Nasara Encore

More Tales from a District Hospital in Tchad

James Appel, MD

To donate to the work going on at the Béré Adventist Hospital, the Moundou Adventist Surgery Center or the Baraka Adventist Hospital Abougoudam visit:

www.ahiglobal.org or www.tchaddoc.com

Scriptures quoted are from the World English Bible, which is a public domain, modern English Bible based on the American Standard Version. For more information visit www.ebible.org

You can obtain additional copies of this book by visiting: www.createspace.com/5710959

Rear cover photo courtesy of Scott Guptil.

Cover design by James Appel, MD

Contact the author at appeltwin1@gmail.com

In Memory of Kaleb Roberts...

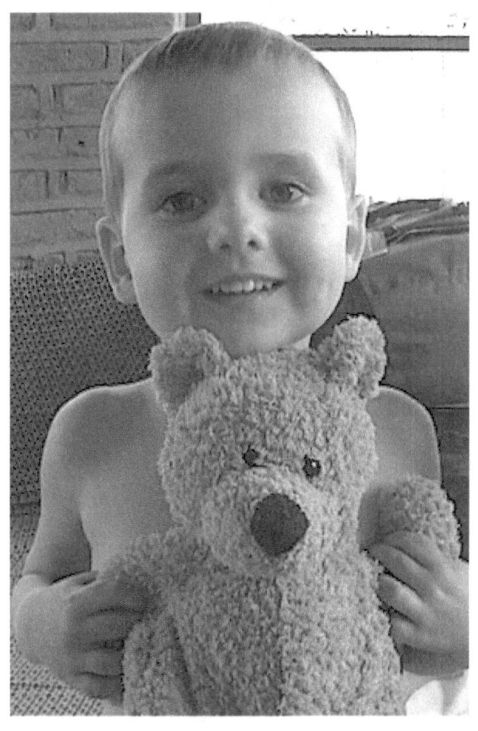

"But we don't want you to be ignorant, brothers, concerning those who have fallen asleep, so that you don't grieve like the rest, who have no hope."

1 Thessalonians 4:13

Also by James Appel, MD:

Nasara: Dispatches from a district hospital in Tchad

https://www.createspace.com/3586897

Children of the East: The spiritual heritage of Islam in the Bible

https://www.createspace.com/3603603

Messiah: The Jesus of the Qur'an and the Gospels

https://www.createspace.com/4129167

Ebola-iculous: A physician encounters the Ebola capital of the world

https://www.createspace.com/5031956

Contents

Introduction

This book is the sequel to my first book, *Nasara: Dispatches from a District Hospital in Tchad.* Both books are mostly written from blogs I sent out over the years that I worked at the Béré Adventist Hospital in the rural south of the Republic of Tchad. I wrote because I was compelled to write. I needed to write to survive. It was my therapy. Thanks to that therapy I am still living and working in Tchad, though not in Béré. But that is another story that remains to be told.

The first book describes my arrival in Tchad, the difficulties of reviving an abandoned district hospital in the bush of one of the world's poorest countries, my falling in love and marrying a Danish nurse volunteer, and my various blundering adventures of living in a foreign culture and facing death almost daily in my patients, friends and colleagues.

This book is the natural continuation of that never-ending story of poverty, suffering, and death and how I dealt with all my failures and inabilities to face it and deal with it along with some of the miraculous successes that came along unexpectedly.

I tried to be as honest as I could and gloss nothing over...after all it was my psychotherapy...I hope and pray it may give insight and meaning to some and inspire others...

N'Djamena 23rd of April, 2017

James Appel, MD

2007

23 January 2007

Nightmares

I wake up with a start. It's 3:26am. The nightmares are back. They always take a different form with the same theme. I'm running from some nameless terror. I have to hide. I am almost found a million times and then...I can tell I'm about to be discovered...and I wake up with my heart pounding in my earplug-filled ears.

The headaches continue. When I'm doing something I'm fine. Just a little nagging in the background. But when I try to relax, a constriction along the top of my neck, through the base of my skull encircles its grasping tentacles around to my throbbing eyes forcing me to want to drink a ton of water and sleep.

My eyes are heavy and my throat is sore. I feel almost desperate for sleep. But there's a lurking fear that when I lie down, I won't be able to rest anyway. So I watch a movie, read a book, or wander around puttering till the inevitable stop of the generator forces me to hit the sack to try and stop my meandering attempts at distraction.

Finally, I lie down. The mattress is soft, yet firm. The pillow is perfect. The bed is long enough for my 6'5" frame to stretch out comfortably in any direction, even when sharing it with a beautiful Dane. I start off with the illusion of falling asleep immediately. Something I long and pray for. It doesn't come. Instead come the slow, persistent, building memories from the day's work, strategies, plans, ideas...anything and everything to keep me from sleeping.

Above all, it's the thoughts of what I should've, could've, would've done. Working at a small bush hospital in sub-saharan Africa as the only physician leaves plenty of fuel for that fire.

I should've cut an episiotomy sooner. The baby was already stressed. Sure it's heart beat was fine. But the 14 year old mom had been in labor on that small pelvis for too long. If I'd only got him out a few minutes earlier he might of made it. It was so close. Why did his heart have to beat so long? Why didn't he ever take a breath?

Why did I even attempt that tendon release? It wasn't life threatening. He'd lived with it for years already. Sure it was painful and made it hard to walk, but I probably just made it worse. I'm way out of my league.

If I'd recognized that meningitis a day sooner instead of only treating his malaria, maybe that little girl would've lived. She made it a couple of days as it was. I'm sure we did everything: IV fluids, glucose, steroids, appropriate antibiotics. What more could we have done?

I should've done a classical incision on that woman with the transverse lie and arm sticking out. If so she wouldn't have torn into both uterine arteries. Sure we managed to control the bleeding, but we almost lost her. What if I'd just done it right the first time?

Did I speak too harshly to the boy with the amputation? His wound had almost healed when he left against medical advice. When he came back with a huge infection needing a higher amputation, I could've spoken more gently. Maybe he would've actually stayed...is he still alive?

How could I have thought it was an ectopic pregnancy? My ultrasound skills suck. An unnecessary operation on a woman with a normal intrauterine pregnancy. I could've saved myself the trouble and her a dangerous procedure.

Is the medical student having a good experience? Should I let him do more? Or less? Is he feeling too overwhelmed with the responsibility? Have I dumped too much on him?

Are Israel and Paul overworked? They are volunteer nurses after all. I want them to have a good time so they'll encourage others to come. Am I assigning them too many night shifts? Do they get tired of my calling them to help with all the surgeries?

Will the work at the hospital ever slow down? We seem to just be getting busier and busier as our staff continues to dwindle and I remain the only doc. I can't even begin to count the surgeries I've done since coming back a few days ago: three to four a day with many minor procedures. The waiting room outside under the mango tree has been constantly packed. There are no beds available in the hospital. People are sleeping outside, their mosquito nets strung from branches of trees. The nurses can't even walk inside at night. Relatives are sleeping on every available floor space including under the beds.

Images flash through my semi-conscious brain: amniotic fluid squirting onto my face as I cut into the uterus to rescue an infant; my fingers push and pull around a tense hydrocele breaking apart the small fibers attaching it to the scrotum with the sound like tearing cardboard; a hernia bulges in and out with the patients breathing as I grab firm fascia and poke through with a needle to close that moving masse inside where it belongs; with a small poke, pus bulges out and flows down the back of the throat like a stream of lava as I quickly suction back and forth on the anesthetized HIV-positive wife of the local chief; moans and babbling float across my brainwaves from a million Tchadians waking up from Ketamine nightmares; the baby's head rolls around despite the firm grasp of Paul as I chase a splinter across his cornea trying to dig it out gently with an 18 gauge needle; gurgles and bad breath roll up at me from an alcoholic desperately wishing he had a bowl of rice wine to assuage his pounding head from the beating he got last night while drunk; urine dribbles onto the ground from a foley bag only partially closed.

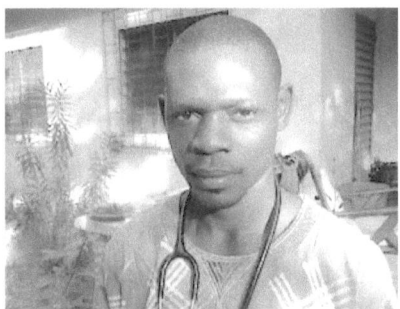

Paul

Words in Arabic, Nangjéré and French wind themselves around my thoughts as I relive my frustration at only being able to communicate on the level of a child. My deep desire to learn Arabic and Nangjéré clashes with feeling so overwhelmed that whenever I have a break I just want something to temporarily distract me.

Finally, I fall asleep, and the nightmare begins...until I jolt awake at 3:26am. My throat is sore, my lips are dry. I grope for a flashlight and take a drink of water in the bathroom. I turn off the light, roll onto my back, try to sink into the mattress. A flashlight appears outside the window rapidly followed by a rap on the metal door. I unplug my ears, grab my headlamp, pull on some shorts and a t-shirt and go to see Clarice and David.

There is a woman in her 10th pregnancy on an oxytocin drip to strengthen her labor. She has been completely dilated for three hours without delivering. I change into scrubs, find my keys, head to the operating room, snatch up the oft-used disposable hand-pump vacuum assist device and head to Labor and Delivery.

I put on gloves and examine the woman. The head is high up but there seems to be room. I wet the vacuum extractor and slide it in over the baby's crown. The woman has a strong contraction. I pump up the vacuum and slowly pull. The head descends and twists to the left as the eyes, nose and mouth pop out slowly over the perineum. I use the bulb suction to clear the airways, release the vacuum and pull the head down to free up the anterior shoulder. Soon comes the squirt of a slimy child, arms and legs firmly contracting, already wanting to scream his anger at the world. We quickly dry the newborn off and wrap her up against the cold. The placenta follows quickly. There are no lacerations and no bleeding. The uterus is firm as a rock.

I go home hoping that for at least of few hours of nightmare-free sleep...

25 January 2007
Unexpected

Yeah, I was tired, but I certainly didn't expect things to turn out that way. I'm still trying to figure it out. But, with our lack of staff and equipment, I'm afraid it's doomed to remain a mystery. I just hope we can do something to change conditions so it doesn't happen again.

It started yesterday. We have been even busier than usual, especially in surgery. We just did our 50th operation of the month yesterday and there's still a week to go in the month.

I had thought the day would be relatively easy. I'd only remembered scheduling a couple of orchiectomies and the excision of an abdominal wall mass. But when I finally got to the operating room at around 11:30am, I found that the first and second cases were both hernias. I don't know how that happened as I've been trying to schedule as many surgeries as possible for next week when a visiting surgeon, Dr. Warren Dekraay, will give me a little break.

I'm already tired having done seven ultrasounds, multiple outpatient consults and a meeting with our HIV patients on anti-retroviral therapy. Contributing to my fatigue is the fact that I was up till midnight the night before operating on a ruptured ectopic pregnancy.

I quickly do the hernias and two orchiectomies. In between, I follow up lab results and see more outpatients. Then, things get a little out of control.

The next surgical patient is a woman with an abdominal mass that is mobile and apparently not fixed to the muscles or anything. There is kind of a peak to it with a little ulceration through the skin. I cut in and pop out six firm fibromas.

Then she starts bleeding like crazy.

She has high blood pressure and every little skin artery shoots out a geyser, spraying everything in sight. I compress the blood vessels as best I can as I call for more hemostat clamps. The cavity is so big and deep I have to excise more skin and open it more to get to find and clamp off all the bleeders. By the time we are done the whole floor, bed, and drapes, as well as our scrubs are covered with the sticky red stuff.

Now it's 3:00pm. I should be going home, but a nomad man has just brought in his wife. She was operated on at another hospital four months ago. Now for two days she hasn't passed gas or stool and vomits all the time. Her belly is distended with absent bowel sounds. She has a bowel obstruction. I send her husband off to pay for the surgery. Meanwhile, the evening nursing team comes to tell me there's a young lad who fell out of a tree and has an open fracture.

Another nurse comes to tell me about a patient we operated on eight days ago for a hernia who's referred from the Bao health center. The reference sheet says he has a strangulated hernia from an "operation badly practiced" at the "Béré BAPTIST Hospital". Interesting, I didn't know there was another hospital here in Béré! I go to examine him and find he has a pretty impressive scrotal hematoma but no hernia. The hernia wound is healing well. When I enter the room, he starts writhing in exaggerated agony. Unfortunately, he'll have to wait.

I go see the boy. His elbow has somehow dislocated and come through the skin of the inside of his elbow without fracturing. The nerve is stretched tense over the exposed joint surface of the humerus. His circulation is intact. He also has a closed distal radio-ulnar fracture dislocation. I take him to surgery as the first priority. What I don't do—

and I'll regret this later—is perform a full physical examination. I also don't check his vital signs.

In surgery I flush out the wound with three liters of irrigation fluid while our medical student, Jamie, and Israel pull the arm in opposite directions. It slowly starts to reduce. With a bend of the arm and a push with my thumb, the humerus enters back into its joint. The elbow bends normally. I rinse out the wound some more and close it up in two layers. I then reduce the wrist and place a cast from hand to above the elbow. The boy does fine with just a minimal dose of diazepam and Ketamine. He is perspiring profusely and his heart rate is elevated, not uncommon with pain and/or Ketamine.

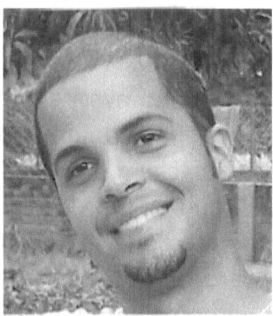

Israel

Since we have neither a post-op recovery room nor enough nurses to staff one, we wheel the boy directly off to pediatrics. I will regret that as well.

We then bring in the nomad woman who ends up having a small bowel obstruction due to two strictures from adhesions caused by her previous surgery. The bowel is dead and requires a resection and anastomosis. As I'm half way through the suturing of the intestine, Clarice enters. I am shocked by what she says.

"The boy is dead"

"Which one?"

"The one with the fracture you just operated on..."

I can't believe it. On further reflection, though, it was inevitable that something like this would happen. In fact, it's a simple miracle that we haven't had more complications or deaths following surgery.

We have become a reference center for people from hundreds of miles around yet our facilities are pathetically inadequate. We have no cardiac monitor. Our pulse oximeter has been broken for over six months. Our large autoclave caught on fire months ago. Our two small autoclaves were fried last week. Now we are sending our instruments an hour away to Kélo to be sterilized.

We only have one operating room which is crammed packed with all our supplies since we have no supply room leaving it difficult to clean properly. We have to walk through the instrument sterilization room to get to the operating room. We have one prep room also stocked from floor to ceiling with supplies. We have no place for patients to change or shower which means a lot of filth gets tracked into the operating room.

We have no post-op recovery room which means patients get dumped on the wards to wake up from anesthesia in the midst of all the other patients. Often, there is only one nurse for all the hospitalized patients who can't possibly give the attention needed to the post-op patients. This means we depend on family members to alert us of problems. This time, it is too late.

What was the cause of the boy's death? Impossible to determine now, especially without an autopsy. However, the real cause is an overworked under-equipped staff and hospital. We need at least one more physician and several more nurses. We also really need a new operating block with at least two operating rooms, a prep room, a post-op recovery room, a dressing room, an instrument sterilization room, and a supply room.

Of course God always helps us in our weaknesses, which is why we've been able to operate successfully on so many with only rare complications. However, if we have the means to improve things and don't, I think God also will hold us accountable for that one day.

Unfortunately, one young boy will not have another chance in this life.

29 January 2007
...You Might Be a Tchadian

If when pregnant the only thing you really crave is dried fish...

If your idea of clean is a well swept dirt yard...

If when the temperature falls below 80 degrees you dust off your parka...

If you've ever traveled to the big city on top of a loaded dump truck...

If you've ever sold a chicken to pay your medical bill...

If you've ever ridden bareback on a cow...

If you refuse to take your horse into the river for fear he'll become a hippo...

If you've ever had to cut a fishing trip short because you got bit in the butt by a hippo...

If you've ever given birth in a rice field...

If you've ever been evacuated to the hospital on a motorcycle...

If you've ever tried to deliver a baby at home who came out hand first...

If your mama's ever slapped you for crying during birth pains...

If you've ever fixed a leaky pipe with an inner tube...

If you've ever fallen out of a mango tree while eight months pregnant...

If your dad took multiple wives to have more workers for his rice field...

If you've ever done surgery without a high school diploma...

If you drink hot tea when it's 130 degrees out...

If you speak more than five obscure languages...

If you're an adult and you've never opened a car door before...

If you've ever thought a cement mixer was an airplane...

If you've ever opened a bottle of Coke with your teeth...

If it's ever taken you two days to travel 42km...

If you've ever repaired a flat tire with needle and thread...

If you've ever packed a car rack higher than the car itself...

If you've ever carried more than your body weight balanced on your head...

If you've ever strapped a baby to your back with a piece of cloth...

If you've ever filled up your gas tank using an old wine bottle, a piece of old hose and a dirty sock...

If you grow gourds on the roof of your house...

If you've ever plowed a field by hand while talking on a cell phone...

If you've ever brought your child to church naked...

If you've ever ridden a motorcycle with an eyeshade over your mouth...

If you've ever paid tithe at church with a goat...

If no one stares when you dress your baby boy in hot pink...

If you've ever talked to your administrator while holding his hand...

If you think nothing of exposing your female breasts but are scandalized by not covering your hair...

If you've ever attended class under a mango tree...

If you've ever broken your arm falling off an ox cart...

If you know more than one person who's been gored by a bull...

If you've ever been thrown in prison for casting a spell on someone...

If you've ever sued someone for killing your pig...

If you've ever killed a rat by stepping on it...

If you've ever barbecued a bat...

If you've ever fixed a radiator with chewing gum...

If when your child has a sore throat you amputate his uvula...

If you feel like an honored guest when you're served soda pop...

If you've ever shared the highway with a herd of longhorns...

If you think all white people look alike...

...YOU MIGHT BE A TCHADIAN!

19 February 2007
Panic

I wake up in a panic. Did I ever really sleep? I'm not sure. Yet, I'm not really awake either. I'm in that gray zone between the netherworld and reality. I Feel the desperation rising within me. Images of the day's surgeries well up along with a nebulous, all-pervading fear that gnaws deep down. It is a fear put into words earlier in the day by Dr. Warren:

"James, I don't know how you're going to be able to handle it when I'm gone. It's just too much."

A retired surgeon, Warren arrived at the end of January. I was excited. I was sure that I would have a break and be able to catch up on so much other stuff I'd let slip by in January. I had reached the breaking point with our 71 surgeries in the first month of 2007, but now, with the arrival of a real surgeon, I was sure that things were on the up swing. Maybe I'd have time for a little exercise: shoot some hoops, go to the river for a swim, ride the horses, jog a little, you know, some leisurely activities having nothing to do with the hospital.

I even hoped that while I was at work I'd have a chance to relax, really follow the inpatients well, have some in depth outpatient visits. You know, be a real doctor for once, not just someone scrambling around to try and do the minimum possible to save as many of the masses that came from all over the country to the one hospital still functioning and still affordable.

I was wrong. Dead wrong.

Warren arrived on Sunday. On Monday, he did two hernias, a hysterectomy and a nephrectomy. I saw 50 inpatients and 28 outpatients, and did six ultrasounds. Then, we all got called in at midnight for a perforated duodenal ulcer that needed to be intubated and resuscitated in a difficult anesthesia case.

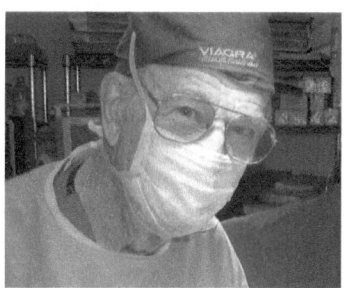
Warren

While Warren operated I was bagging the patient and telling Paul what drugs to give to keep the man alive. We managed to save his live for a few days before he succumbed to who knows exactly what since we have no electrolyte or chemistry panels in our lab and no intensive care.

Then, things started to get really bad.

First, the big autoclave has been out for months waiting for parts. Then, within the week prior to Warren's arrival, both small autoclaves got fried. Then, the generator went out leaving us without water or power. We had a small generator given us by the Shanks, friends working at the Koza Adventist Hospital in Cameroon. That at least allowed us a little light, suction and a monitor in the operating room. However, Warren, at the age of 74, has been forced to work without air conditioning in the ever-increasing Tchadian hot season.

And work he has. In three weeks, counting today, he's done 55 surgeries. Many of them have been complicated like the man with a redundant small bowel cyst, a C-section with eight liters of ascites and an ovarian cyst the size of a soccer ball. He's also done many hysterectomies and some cases of osteomyelitis. Of course, there's always plenty of hernias and hydroceles as well.

The lab then ran out of power. We hooked everything up in reverse (since the small generator is 110V and the hospital is wired for 220V) so that the lab battery could charge and they can run things off the inverter. I thought we had it all fool proofed, but they managed to fry a microscope bulb and the hematocrit machine. Now, we can't even check a hemoglobin. Instead, we rely entirely on the color of the conjunctiva to decide if a person needs to be transfused. Modern day medicine at it's best.

We've adapted. We've borrowed a 220V generator from the Local Health District office to pump water every few days. We continue to operate with the small 110V generator. I see about twice as many outpatients as normal. Plus the number of inpatients has increased as we get more well-known and we do more surgery. We've borrowed a stand up autoclave that takes six hours to sterilize. We use either a kerosene or propane stove stuck underneath trying to heat it up since we have neither an electrical heating element nor the power source to run one if we did.

For the moment we have no accountant. We've given him a leave of absence to try and find money to pay off the $1200 he stole from the hospital. We've also been without our administrator as André has been in N'Djamena for most of the month trying to get medicines from the central pharmacy. We've run out of even basic medicines like Bactrim and Flagyl. We haven't had a new urine collection bag in months. We've been re-washing the old ones and using feeding tube bags as well. As a result, I've had to hand all administrative issues as well.

All the nurses are working themselves to the bone at the same time. What would we do without our two student missionary nurses, Paul and Israel? We've been blessed with our new, half-deaf nurse, Abel. He's not above getting down and dirty to assist on surgeries, clean up the blood and guts, wash the instruments, and stay till sundown almost every day. The Ministry of Health has also just assigned two new nurses to our hospital.

God always gives us just enough to get by.

And then there's today which should have been a relaxed Sunday with no scheduled surgeries. It starts with a bloody C-section for uterine rupture which ends up in a hysterectomy. The patient needs four blood transfusions as we have difficulty controlling the bleeding. Then a case of osteomyelitis of the tibia followed by an incarcerated hernia that comes in during the C-section.

Since eating a few hash browns for breakfast I don't eat again until I grab some cold pasta late in the evening. Now, panic sets in as I think about Dr. Warren's soon departure. How will I handle it? And more importantly, what will happen to the hospital and health care in the region when Sarah and I go on vacation March 11? And when both Paul and Israel leave at about the same time?

More importantly, how will my body handle this stress? I can't even sleep. I spend my nights tossing and turning, begging God with racking sobs to intervene. It's been too much for too long and the burden is just getting heavier. Is God not listening? Or has God been calling someone to help but that person is not listening? All I know is that I'm not going to last much longer without some kind of intervention.

13 February 2007
Jaws & Bladders

Her face is so swollen it is all but unrecognizable. Her right eye is completely shut. Blood caked in streaks and dotted lines runs from her lower lip, down her chin, around a large gash under her jaw and across her neck where it has spattered her shirt with dark maroon patches like a painted mustang. Out of her left ear and nose dribbles an oily, blood-tinged liquid. Patches of bloody cotton stuffed haphazardly into her left ear attempt to control the flow.

She is awake, alert and not afraid despite being small for an eight year old. Her father has brought her all the way from Kélo on a motorcycle after she fell from a mango tree that afternoon.

It is Sunday night and I've had a long, busy day at the hospital.

She opens her mouth to reveal a cut inside along the gums leading to a visible mandible fracture. Most of the teeth on the right have been knocked out except one molar on the top, a split molar on the bottom and four of her front teeth, all caused by an addiction to mangos. What can I say? I'm guilty myself.

As I have them prepare for immediate surgery, Lona and Rahama, the nurses on duty, ask me to see an old man who can't pee. Lona tried to pass a foley catheter but was unable to get it into the bladder. I walk into labor & delivery where they've placed him and see a sobering sight.

A wizened, almost blind man in his 70's is squatting on one of the delivery beds with a wrap half covering his manhood. His chest is bare, sunken and twisted. His scrawny arms still reveal what was once a wiry, tough man. Blood is smeared all over the table, the wrap, and the man's groin where partially clotted blood drips from his urethra.

His bladder is swollen halfway to his belly button. I stick a gloved finger up his rectum and confirm a grossly enlarged prostate. He begs to be taken home so he can die. I explain that we will operate on him first thing in the morning and that he won't die. He refuses. We leave the sons to reason with him while Israel, Paul, Sarah and I take the small girl to the operating room.

Sarah administers the general anesthesia and I attempt to wire her jaw. I take a steel suture and pass it around the base of her only two molars on the right. I twist them together leaving a tail that I then twist together with the molar's twin to bring the jaw together in a functional position. I repeat the process with the front teeth. It's sketchy, but is sort of working.

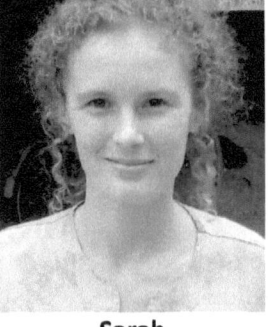

Sarah

I then open up our internal, maxillofacial fixation tray and enlarge the wound between her lower lip and chin to expose the fracture. I drill four small holes through a small compression plate, measure the depth of the holes, select the appropriate sized screws and carefully screw them in with a hand screwdriver. Just like I learned in carpentry class!

We wash out the wounds well. I close some of them and Israel closes the rest. She also has a probable basilar skull fracture causing the cerebrospinal fluid to come out her nose and ears. I put her on a broad spectrum antibiotic for a week. A few days later the swelling is almost gone. Her pain is controlled with ibuprofen and Tylenol. After a week the leaking from her nose and ears has stopped and she goes home.

Meanwhile, I come out of the operating room to find that the man with the enlarged prostate is at the gate and would've been home already if the night watchman hadn't blocked his leaving.

As I walk up to him under the starry Tchadian sky a huge part of me wants to just yell at him for being so stupid and let him go home to die. He refuses to wait for the morning saying he'll die before then.

Nasara Encore

The air is cool and I am tired. It's 11pm already. But, an unfortunately rare thought enters my head: what if it was my dad? My grandpa? Me? What would I want done?

I offer to operate right now. After much discussion and suspicious glances thrown my way by the old man, his sons convince him.

We carry him to the operating room, prep him and give him a spinal anesthetic. I scrub my already well scrubbed hands. I'm almost in a dream, a moment frozen in time as my hands go through the automatic ritual of nails, fingers, hands, wrists to the elbows that has been drilled into me. It's a comforting and important ritual.

I open the operating room door with my back, elbows out and hands up. I grab a towel, dry my hands slowly and methodically, and drop the towel on the floor. I grab the gown, shake it out and slide my hands through. I'm in another world. I put on my sterile gloves. Then Israel and I place the sterile towels around the lower abdomen of the man and then lay on the drape.

After prayer, I take the scalpel and slice horizontally through the skin right above the symphysis pubis, the same as for a C-section. I cut down to the fascia and just through to the muscle on either side of the mid-line. I take the scissors, spread them under the fascia to detach the muscles and cut to the edges of the skin incision both ways. I grab and lift the fascia with clamps. Then, with my fingers and scissors I separate the muscles from the fascia first superiorly and then inferiorly. I split the muscles with a clamp, insert my fingers and pull the muscles apart. Israel inserts retractors and I open the bladder with the scalpel in a vertical incision. Israel uses the suction tubing to sop up the fountain of urine that pours out. I extend the incision with the scissors.

Israel sucks out all the urine and then pulls the wound open with the retractors. I find the posterior part of the prostate and make a nick with the scalpel. Then we pull out all clamps and retractors and I stick my finger into the bladder, find the small incision and push into the mucosa around the prostate and then sweep around the prostate, shelling it out. Blood pours into the bladder as I lift out the trophy.

Paul inserts a small urethral dilator from below, I attach a heavy suture to the dilator, and Paul pulls it out the urethra. He then ties the suture to a large foley catheter which is then guided into the bladder around the false track. Paul inserts 30ml of water and yanks the foley down into the hole that used to have the prostate.

Israel and I close the bladder, fascia and skin while Paul attaches the irrigation tubing to the three way foley catheter as bloody fluids start coming out into the urine bag.

The next day, the patient is pleasantly surprised to find himself still alive. I'm surprised to find out he lives right next to the hospital. He's even more surprised to find out a week later that he is going home in very good condition with normal urine function. The only draw back is that he has to suffer through a large indwelling catheter for another week.

"Lapia, merci beja," He smiles, grabs my hand with both his and repeats over and over "Lapia, lapia, lapia..."

18 March 2007

Gwame

I strip down to my underwear and half-walk, half run down the sandy slope and plunge into the coolness of the river. The hot season is upon us and nothing is cool here except the river. The harmattan winds blow hot dust and wind off the Sahara leaving the Sun a well defined, somewhat darkened orb in a murky sky.

Sarah, Israel and I have brought our two volunteer resident physicians, Aimee and Jennifer out here on horseback. Everyone is hot, dusty and sweaty but I'm the only one to take the plunge. I feel invigorated and take long crawl strokes upstream. However, due to the force of the current and my long unused swimming muscles my progress is slow and fatigue comes on fast. Every once in a while I lift my head up for along look ahead. One never knows if there might be hippos!

I pull out of the water and dry off with my shirt. I pull on my pants. Sarah and Israel have disappeared with the two horses. The girls inform me that the horses ran off. Sarah and Israel soon come back with the strays. I grab the single rope attached to the nose bridle, place my left foot in the stirrup and swing up. My butt is already sore from being too long out of the saddle.

We start off in a slow trot. Aimee is riding behind Sarah and Jennifer behind Israel. They are bouncing up and down like jackhammers. It looks painful! They can't really gallop so I spur my horse, Bob, on ahead. The wind whips through my hair as I fly over the dusty trails past the burned fields awaiting the transformation of the next rainy season. There is one field that is surrounded by a two foot high thorn fence and dirt retaining wall where someone is desperately and pathetically trying to grow something. To me it looks like he's growing weeds, or maybe "weed".

A pack of women with huge metal basins covered with brightly colored cloth perched on their heads block my path. I pull in the rein tightly and Bob slows down. At the same time, they realize that a horse is upon them and quickly move to the side. I wave and shout "*Lapia*" and continue on.

I turn around and gallop into the harmattan winds until I rejoin the others and we slowly walk back. At the first house on the outskirts of the village Sarah stops to ask if they have any chickens. They don't have any. Too bad since we were hoping for something special for the going away party for our volunteers.

Just then I see Gwame run up. A cute five year old, he is wearing old shorts, a torn shirt and a huge grin as he stops near my horse with arm outstretched to give me "five". After I slap his hand his tongue pokes out in concentration. He pulls back his palm to smack mine with all his little might.

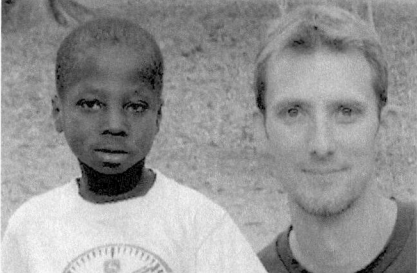
Gwame & James

Hard to believe that less than a year ago he was a cripple with nothing but a lifetime of suffering ahead of him.

In August, thanks to my old friend Troy Dickson and his wife he was sent to Kenya to the Cure Hospital for a life-changing operation. He had what is called "wind swept knees." Both knees were displaced laterally as if a strong wind was blowing them to the side making it almost impossible for him to walk. In fact, when Troy and I first saw him he was also malnourished and covered with scabies from head to toe. Being an identical twin made it even sadder as by looking at his brother we could see what he should be.

Now, radiating joy and health he begs me to lift him up for a horse ride. I reach down and grab him under the armpit and swing his little body into the saddle. His straightened legs easily fall on either side of the horses shoulder and off we go.

We take off in a trot with the neighborhood kids following screaming at the top of their lungs. The permanent grin on Gwame's face threatens to split his ears in two. We come back and chase the other kids all the way into the courtyard of the house. Gwame giggles and chuckles with a contagious hilarity that makes us all feel like nothing could touch us in this moment. We are as free as free can be. Free to rejoice in a miracle, in a transformed life, in the moment.

20 March 2007
Mission

I'm sitting in the dark. The generator has just wound to a halt. A kerosene lamp gives it's warm, but not far-reaching light to an otherwise shadow-filled room. Sarah has gone to N'Djamena to take our Danish medical student, Trine, to the airport for her return to Denmark. It's just me and the guys. I'm sitting at the table in front of the lamp. The cat is playing with my foot as if it were a dead rat. Israel is lying on the couch on the right. Paul is sitting on the couch to the left.

Israel is a nurse from Puerto Rico recently graduated from Southern Adventist University. He is fluent in English and Spanish and already speaks French quite well after only two months. He has taken night shifts where he is the only nurse in the hospital and post-call still comes into help in surgery. He's what you might call a missionary stud.

Not to be left behind is Paul. A Nigerian trained at the Ile-Ife Adventist Hospital, he has had the highest level of nursing training, speaks fluent English, Hausa and Yoruba and has also learned enough French to be very dangerous. Despite not being Adventist and having most of his classmates tell him not to come to some God-forsaken place like Tchad, he has dedicated a year of his life to help his Tchadian brothers.

Both have fearlessly followed Sarah's lead and learned to ride horses the hard way. Both have fallen off their horses at full gallop and lived to tell the tale.

Israel states that if he could have his loans from nursing school paid off he'd gladly spend at least four years in the mission field. But he hasn't found any way to do it.

Paul brings up a problem at Ile-Ife where he trained. He literally begs me if there is anything that can be done to bring in specialist physicians, especially surgeons. They desperately need a general surgeon, orthopedist or traumatologist as they see so many motor vehicle accidents with mass casualties needing surgical intervention. They also need a neurosurgeon for the same reason: lots of head trauma. If only someone could come and teach their physicians and help them take care of the overwhelming load. Since when does the Third World not really need our help anyway?

Somehow I think in the West we have the idea that since developing countries do have their own doctors and nurses then they should be taking care of their compatriots' needs. But most of third world doctors are in the cities chasing wealth just like their Western colleagues. No one is willing to go out to the small villages and towns. So even in Nigeria, where things are a lot more developed than Tchad, Paul is pleading, "please, we need help!"

Meanwhile, here in Béré, our hospital officially serves a population of 142,000 not counting the thousands who come to us from the outside our health district. I'm the only physician.

There are so many amazing things that I'm getting to experience professionally and spiritually that others should have the chance to share. How much more could we be experiencing if we were a team and not just a burned-out, overworked doctor-nurse team trying desperately to salvage what lives we can from the teeming masses of under-treated people so desperate to find healing that they'll come from miles and miles around to our pathetic hospital just because it's so much better than they can find where they are.

But maybe I'm just tired and needing to vent.

27 May 2007
Crash

Hot air like a Danish sauna blasts up to smack me in the face as I step out the door onto the runway in N'Djamena. Two months have flown by as Sarah and I trekked across Europe from Paris to Denmark to Portugal and then all across the USA from California to Florida to Tennessee. We're back in Tchad, refreshed and not quite prepared for the crushing news soon to be unleashed upon us.

We clear customs without any difficulty. Job and Aimé are waiting outside to take us to the mission house at AIM. We stop on the porch to chat and Sarah asks when Israel, Paul and Dr. Bond will be up with the truck so we can go down to Béré.

Job has seemed strangely distant all evening and now his face exudes his anguish as he tells us the story:

"The truck won't be coming for you...you see, there's been an accident..." Job sits us down and we hear the rest of the story.

Last Saturday, Sarah and I were in the USA chatting with some friends from Africa in the comfort of my cousin's house in Chattanooga, Tennessee. Meanwhile, back in Béré, Noel, André and the rest were preparing to leave church when a raging man broke in violently and tried to attack our chaplain. Before he could reach Noel, he was restrained and Noel was quickly ushered into a back room. The man was identified as the son of one of our janitors. After the would be assailant was convinced to return home, Noel continued on to the hospital to see the patients.

However, unbeknownst to the rest of us, the man followed Noel. When it was seen that he was heading for the hospital, the gatekeeper quickly locked the gate and Noel hid inside. The man jumped the fence, now armed with a knife. As he ran around hunting for Noel, the hospitalized patients' caregivers fought him off with sticks, brooms, and anything else they could get their hands on to keep him away from Noel.

Finally, André was able to contact the gendarmes who came and subdued him, but not before he had stabbed and destroyed one of the two air conditioners in the operating rooms. The man was taken to prison. He struggled so hard he managed to break one of the jail doors before finally being locked up.

That same day, it was discovered that our Accountant, Ganota, who we'd just fired for embezzlement, had managed to sneak into the garage and steal five bicycles, several large cooking pots and a generator. Somehow, he'd broken in the back door and been carrying things off little by little.

These items were left by patients as collateral for their hospital debts. We only found out about the thefts when a former patient came back to reclaim his bike only to find it wasn't there. André and Pierre went quickly to the market and found Ganota loading the stuff on to a bus. He planned to ship it to his home town of Léré.

Pierre and André were able to recover all the lost items, but Ganota managed to slip away into the crowd. A warrant was immediately put out on Ganota but he was never caught. Ganota's wife immediately began to pack up to return to Léré herself to be with her relatives.

Monday, Sarah and I headed back down to Florida with my parents and my sister Chelsey. The van was pulling a U-Haul trailer with my sisters' college stuff. 20 minutes outside of Chattanooga, Chelsey heard a noise from the back tire. We stopped, but couldn't find anything wrong. When it continued, we were forced to find a mechanic who took the whole wheel off and declared there was nothing wrong.

Shortly after getting back on the freeway, a woman passed us in a car waving her hands and pointing at the trailer. Dad hesitated. We'd had one false warning already. Chelsey looked back and said the trailer's wheel was wobbling. I told Dad to pull over at once. We slowed down quickly and moved over through traffic to the side of the road.

Examining the trailer wheel we found that the bearing had completely disintegrated. The axel was almost completely out from the wheel leaving just a centimeter of axel holding the wheel on. If the wheel had fallen off at full speed, the trailer would've fishtailed causing it to flip taking the van with it. At 75 mph on a crowded interstate there would've been a lot of funerals to attend.

Meanwhile, back in Béré, André agrees to give Ganota's wife a lift to the nearby town of Kélo where she has arranged for some relatives to send her some money. Arriving in Kélo, she finds that Ganota has proceeded her and somehow, despite André's advance warning to the relatives, managed to con the money from them.

The truck is full. André's two year old son, his niece, his mother in law and Ganota's daughter are also inside. Ganota's wife has no money so André decides to drive them all to Pala, half-way to Léré.

On the outskirts of Pala, André hits a stretch of "washboard" road. Suddenly, without warning the car starts to slide and he loses control. Instinctively, he tries to brake resulting in locked wheels which, according to police reports, skid 31 meters veering to the right off the road. When he hits the ditch at the side, the car turns on it's right side just in time to collide with all it's forward momentum into a huge tree trunk.

The roof takes the brunt of the force and is smashed to within inches of the bottom of the back seats, tearing the metal supports on both sides of the windshield off. André slams forward bending the steering wheel 45 degrees with his chest and taking the windshield on the head. He is knocked unconscious. His mother-in-law in the front seat suffers a similar fate.

In the back seat, André's niece and his son are killed instantly. Ganota's wife manages to open her eyes and say a few words to those who quickly pulled everyone from the car before she dies. Ganota's daughter miraculously survives even though being in the completely compressed back seat. She has minimal lacerations on her scalp and some bumps and bruises.

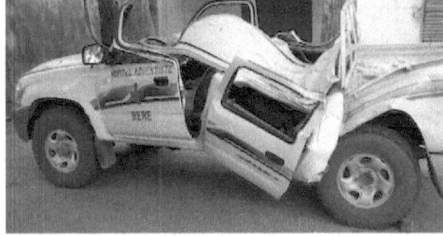

Hilux

The car is virtually unrecognizable despite having no damage to either tires, wheels, chassis or motor. However, the extensive damage to the cabin is sobering as one realizes that no one should have survived that accident.

After hearing the news from Job that first night in N'Djaména sleep is difficult. I toss and turn only to wake up early. We are forced to take public transport. Job accompanies us. We arrive at the chaotic Dembé market. We find a mini-van filled with people and a loaded rack apparently ready to leave. Blessing our good fortune we pay up and sit down to wait for the "one other passenger" that they need in order to leave.

After 15 minutes, the people start to get out of the van until it is empty. Then, they start to unload some suspiciously light sacks until there is virtually nothing on top. We have been duped and are forced to wait an hour and a half until they really find enough passengers. By this time, it's already after 2pm and we have a long journey ahead of us.

On the way to Pala, Sarah and I are crammed in the very back seat. My seat has no back, only the rear window to rest my head against. We share the seat with a Tchadian woman and her shy child who plays incessantly with a noise-making toy cell-phone. Sarah tries to discourage him by poking him every time the cell phone makes a sound. It doesn't work.

In front of us, as the journey progresses, I watch unfold one of the most unusual and astounding things I have seen in my three plus years in Tchad: public affection between a man and wife. I am mesmerized by their intimacy. They actually seem to enjoy each others company leaning their heads in closely to share secrets. Her arm rests lovingly on his shoulder. He casually loops his arm around hers. As night approaches, their heads lean in and touch as they alternately rest and share intimate moments in their own little world. She has the traditional muslim head covering and he, while not dressed in Arabic robes, is obviously a firm believer as he steps out to pray with the others as the van takes breaks at all the appropriate prayer times.

In order to appreciate the magnitude of this, one has to have lived in Africa and seen the total separation of the sexes. Men and women eat apart, socialize only with their own gender and come together only in private for making children. One may see gruff soldiers walking down the street hand in hand all the time, but rarely will one see a girl and boy or man and woman making even this most minimal of public gestures of affection.

One time, before a trip that Sarah was making, as I was hugging her good bye I saw that Pierre and his wife had arrived. Pierre was going to accompany Sarah, so to tease him I told him, "Pierre, this is how we say *au revoir* in my culture." He replied that it was a good custom and he was willing to try it. As he moved toward his wife, she began to laugh nervously, quickly got up and moved rapidly out of reach. Pierre would have to wait for another day to try that new cultural experience!

We arrive late in Kélo and have to wait another hour for the bus to Pala. We finally leave a little after 10:00pm only to be stopped by the gendarmes at the exit of the village. The route is barred and they say that no one can travel after 10:00pm so we might as well just settle down and sleep till morning. The driver turns off the van and everyone sits there stunned. I feel a little nervous, but decide I should try something.

I cautiously approach the soldiers in the dark and greet them. Each of them is carrying an AK47. I introduce myself as the doctor from the Béré Adventist Hospital just down the road. I explain the situation with André and the accident and how I'd like to see him tonight so I can return to Béré in the morning. Otherwise, I point out, the hospital will be without a doctor.

"I heard there's a national strike going on and the Kélo hospital is closed." I add. "Wouldn't that be tragic if one of your relatives got sick, decided to go the the only hospital around that's open—in Béré—and find that there wasn't a doctor there? I wonder if there's any way you can help us?"

The guards tell me to come over and sit on the bench with them. I get up from where I'd been squatting on the ground in front of them and sit down. They call up their superior and explain the situation. After a few minutes, they call over the driver and tell him to get his passengers in and get on the road. We make it to Pala a little after midnight where we stretch out on woven mats on the ground to sleep. Mosquitos buzz around my head in the dark. There are no lights on in the entire hospital as my brain tries to wrap itself around the fact that only 36 hours ago I was in Paris.

C'est la vie au Tchad!

10 June 2007
Sight to the Blind

The wizened little Arab grandpa has already been in the hospital for awhile. He arrived at the end of my vacation and was operated on for a hydrocele. Then he was re-hospitalized for a urinary tract infection with urinary retention. He has come back now for the third time with urinary retention once again. He has an enlarged prostate and I schedule him for surgery tomorrow.

I approach his bed in the semidarkness of an overcast day. There are no lights without the generator. At his side is another old Arab with a gap-toothed smile revealing gnarly teeth pointing in all the directions of the compass. Another elderly robed muslim hangs out quietly in the corner next to what appears to be a middle aged woman. She wears a brightly colored green dress with puffy sleeves. A shawl draped lazily over her head partially covers the small leather fetish pouches dangling haphazardly from a thick leather cord around her neck. She is breast feeding a child cradled absentmindedly in her right arm.

"As-salaamu aleikum," I start the long greeting process in Arabic.

When we have finished the ritual the family tells me that suddenly, last night, the patient became totally blind. Also, he has been vomiting since yesterday despite his intravenous malaria treatment. I examine him and confirm that he no vision in either eye.

I can think of no medical explanation for it but plenty of spiritual ones.

"Ibliss or one of the djinns has blinded him," I explain. "Only by praying to Allah, the one true God, can he be healed."

They all nod expectantly and gather around with hands outstretched, palms up ready to receive baraka (blessing) from Allah. I pray in the same way with my arms and hands in the appropriate position.

As I finish they all smile and demonstrate a faith I can only marvel in. They have complete confidence now that Allah's will will be done.

None of us are surprised the next morning to come and find his vision completely restored. They all just smile, hold their hands out while looking up and saying "*Al hamdullilah.*"

27 June 2007
Moto-taxi

It feels good to be on the road again. I never thought that a trip to N'Djamena would be something to look forward to, especially without my own car. However, after practically never leaving the hospital in the month I've been back in Tchad, it's good to be going somewhere.

Besides, it's a relatively cool morning, the desert is starting to be transformed into the green African Sahel and I'm on the back of a *moto-taxi* with the wind blasting my face bringing tears to my eyes. The humid, fragrant smell of freshly rained-on earth and grass rushes into my brain bringing back memories of calmer times.

Sarah and I are accompanying our Swiss volunteer, Esther, to the airport and then hope to bring back enough medicines and supplies to make it through the rainy season when the road to Béré gets really bad. Esther's *moto-taxi* was the first to be off, followed by Sarah's. They are no where in sight.

The overcast sky starts to lift as a few rays of sun pierce the clouds. The red clay road already has a few mud holes that the *moto-taxi* man zigzags through like a professional slalom skier. It seems that my driver is a little more aggressive than most and I notice that we seem to be accelerating even more than usual. We skirt the potholes and dodge the goats, chickens, bikes, kids and women carrying goods to market on their heads. Our speed steadily increases.

I'm trying not to worry about what will happen to my helmet-less head if we slip in the slimy clay or hit a hole or something. We go faster and faster. I notice the taxi man fiddling with a cable coming out of the handlebar. It hits me: the accelerator is stuck. He wiggles, pushes, twists and turns the cable as our velocity steadily increases. I now truly feel like I'm in the Olympic downhill as we carom at ever increasing angles in our now deadly slalom course.

At about the same moment as I ask myself why he doesn't just turn the engine off I see him reach for the ignition. My gaze follows his hand to where the key should be. There's nothing there! Apparently, the bouncing of the dirt road has shook the key out of the ignition. I see the key flapping in the breeze attached to the handlebar by a cell phone SIM card and a small wire.

We aren't slowing down.

All my hopes rest on the coordination of this stranger as the key plays keep away with his desperately grasping fingers. Finally, he has it. Now, as he continues careening around holes driving with one hand, he plays target practice with his other trying to fit the key into the jiggling, wiggling, shaking ignition.

The key enters and is quickly turned to off. The *moto* slowly decreases it's velocity as we cruise around the mud holes and finally come to rest, like Noah's ark after the flood, on the side of the road.

My taxi man apparently is also a mechanic. He pulls off a makeshift, crudely welded tool, uses his hand as a hammer and hits the tool against the cover of where the accelerator cable enters the engine until it slowly unscrews. He fiddles with the cable that had some gunk in it keeping it from releasing. When he's satisfied it's back to "normal" we get back on and continue on our way.

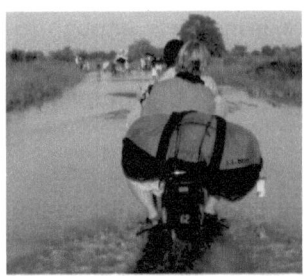

Moto-taxi

Now, I'm starting to feel the uncomfortableness of wearing a heavy backpack that is forced up onto my shoulder blades by Esther's hard suitcase that has been strapped vertically on the back of the *moto* with some strips of old inner-tube.

About eight kilometers from Kélo—35 from Béré—the back wheel starts to make some serious grinding noises. We stop again. The bearing is shot. We get back on and start to move forward at about 10 km/hour. It feels and sounds as if the wheel could fall off at any time.

Then we run out of gas. Coincidentally it seems, at the same time I notice that all the clouds have disappeared, the sun has moved higher in the sky, the humidity has increased and I'm starting to seriously sweat— even before we start to push the *moto* the last three kilometers to Kélo.

Despite the weight of the *moto* and the grinding of the back wheel, we still manage to pass a lot of people on foot. My hands grip the top of the suitcase and my thighs start to burn. As the women whisper and giggle to see a tall, skinny white dude passing them pushing a *moto*, I start to wonder if my out of shape body will last for three kilometers.

Miraculously, 45 minutes later we arrive on the outskirts of Kélo.

My taxi man calls another *moto* taxi over who he says he'll take me across town for 500 CFA. I laugh and tell him I didn't just arrive here yesterday. I'd already agreed to pay 3000 CFA to go to the bus station and if my *moto* can't make it then it's up to my taxi man to arrange other transport. The crowd that has gathered laughs in approval. The two taxi men smile begrudgingly and work it out among themselves.

Finally, I arrive at the Kélo bus stop, 43 painful kilometers later, only just the beginning of a long journey to the capital.

28 June 2007
A Sad Tale

Sarah comes to wake me up just after I've fallen asleep. It is a Friday night.

"I think I have a patient who needs a symphysiotomy," She says.

I drag myself out of bed trying desperately to sweep the cobwebs from my mind. I'm so adrenaline-depleted after the long day in the operating room that I can barely summon enough reserve to pull on my scrubs, slip on my Crocs and stumble through the moonlit night towards the hospital.

That morning I had taken out two huge prostates from a couple of old Arabs before being called back to the clinic to see a man with a strangulated hernia. We took him immediately to the operating room where I sliced open his groin to reveal a hernia sack the size of a medium size Ziplock filled with stale, bloody inflammatory fluid and a portion of small intestine hanging onto life by its teeth.

As I cut open the internal inguinal ring I watch carefully to see if the dusky intestine will pink up. Slowly, but surely, the tiny capillaries on the glistening intestinal surface start to pump back to life. While the intestine doesn't return completely to normal color it is encouraging enough that I shove it back in the man's belly, repair the hernia in three layers and close the skin.

In the next case, I take out small ovarian cysts on a young woman. Afterwards, I cut out a weird, cystic mass on a three year old boy right below his belly button in the midline.

Tuesday through Thursday had also been brutal with two hysterectomies, a double sided recurrent hernia after a ten year old repair and three c-sections.

One of the c-sections was for a ruptured uterus requiring a hysterectomy. The abdominal wall on the ruptured side was in tatters. I tried to suture it, but despaired of stopping the bleeding for a long time. Another one of the c-sections had an allergic reaction to the lidocaine spinal anesthetic causing her lungs to clamp down and her blood pressure to plummet. Only after intubating her, giving her steroids, adrenaline, bronchodilators and a ton of IV fluids were we able to save her. We then did the C-section pulling out a screaming five kilogram monster of a newborn.

I also took out a prostate the size of a baseball—each of the three lobes would've qualified as prostatic hypertrophy in and of itself.

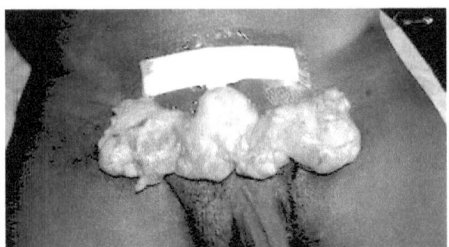

Prostate

So, now, Friday night, I clumsily follow Sarah to the labor and delivery suite. The pregnant girl is in her mid-teens and tiny. Her legs are midget sized. She has to be under 5 feet tall. I learn it's her second pregnancy. Two years ago she had labored at home for days before going to another hospital where they somehow managed to extract the dead fetus. This time, she's been in labor for three days. I feel the belly. It's tender and she has lost her normal uterine contour. A ruptured uterus.

David, the night watchman, calls Siméon and Abel while we start to prepare for surgery. As I attempt to insert the urinary catheter I find it won't pass more than an inch. I check and confirm that the head of the baby is blocking the urinary outflow tract. As I push up the head of the fetus, a gush of urine comes out. Apparently, she had a fistula from her previous long delivery. Her urethra is completely scarred down with urine leaking uncontrollably out of her vagina. We are forced to abandon the urinary catheter.

I place a spinal anesthetic, prep and drape her abdomen, Abel prays and I cut down quickly in a midline incision. Dark blood gushes out as I enter the abdominal cavity. Abel aspirates up the blood with the suction catheter while I pull out the large dead baby. I then gaze at the dark edges of the uterine rupture which look like an exit wound from a shotgun blast.

Fortunately, it's anterior, almost exactly where we would've made our uterine incision for a normal C-section. I trim off the dead muscle and suture up the tear. She should recover fine but will have to come back in a couple of months to have her fistula repaired. In the mean time, she will be incontinent of urine having already tragically and needlessly lost two newborns.

I go back to sleep a little after midnight.

At three, I am woken from an even deeper sleep by my lovely red-headed wife. Again, she brings bad news. Another girl has arrived in labor since this morning. I manage to once more drag myself out of bed and accompany Sarah back to the hospital. She says this girl is from the same village over 40 km away and is practically the same size.

As I enter labor and delivery room I swear this girl is the other girl's twin. However, for this teenager, it is her first pregnancy, the fetal heart beat is still there and her uterus appears intact. Her pelvis is small and the baby's head is completely deformed from trying to be squeezed out a too small opening.

I grab the symphysiotomy tray, inject local anesthetic over her pubic bone, insert a urinary catheter, move the catheter to the side with my left hand inside and cut through the skin down to cartilage with my right hand. I then cut through the fibers from top to bottom until I'm mostly through the pubis, which connects the pelvis together in front.

I then have Sarah and David the night watchman pull her legs out and down effectively opening her pelvis about 3 cm. I attach a hand pump vacuum—a single use item in the USA—that we've used for over a year now. The head descends and a fat, screaming baby comes out less than five minutes later.

I suture up a couple of small vaginal lacerations and the symphysiotomy wound, help mop up the blood and fluids and head home.

Two teenagers, practically twins, but different outcomes based on a simple decision on when to come to the hospital. Same initial presentation but one "twin" has two dead babies, urinary incontinence from a difficult-to-repair fistula, a huge abdominal scar, a recently sutured large tear in her uterus and a long recovery ahead of her with dismal prospects for more children. If she does become pregnant, she will die if she doesn't have a scheduled C-section before boing into labor.

On the other hand, the second "twin" has a healthy newborn, a small pubic scar and can deliver vaginally safely for however many children she and her husband decide to have.

04 July 2007
Death Encore

I'm not even sure what time it is as I stumble like a drunk man trying to walk the line over to the hospital. It has to be after midnight and there is no moon leaving me in blackness like the inside of a cave. Only my dim headlamp briefly lights up the grass on either side of the path like the headlights of a car going in slow motion.

David thanks me for coming and I mumble something in reply. I just can't clear the cobwebs and I didn't even take Benadryl or anything. Maybe it was the four hour surgery earlier on top of three previous ones the same day capped off by learning that the patient died three hours later. While it wasn't a surprise since he'd had intestinal volvulus for over a week, it still is draining.

I come into the ER and see a child. He's panting. His eyes are wide with an almost vacant stare. His belly is swollen and tender. He hasn't pooped or farted since the morning. He needs an operation.

I manage to scribble out some orders. Then I weave my way over to where the night watchman has slung out a thin, lumpy cotton mattress on the cement in front of the clinic. Right before slumping onto the mattress, I tell David to call the operating room team and wake me when the patient is ready.

I collapse. My whole body wants to sink through the mattress and even the cement. As I drift off, I beg God to somehow give me the strength to do this operation.

In what seems like no time, Siméon is shaking me awake. "We're ready."

I wearily get up and enter the surgical suite. A few moments later, I stare at the 18 month old boy lying naked on the blue plastic covering the operating room table. I have a hard time imagining that I'm actually going to shortly be taking a very sharp scalpel and slicing open his belly.

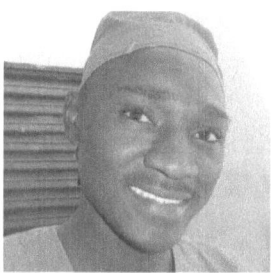

Siméon

When I do, pus comes out in clumps mixed with slippery, inflammatory fluid. We suction and suction all the corners of the abdomen until we've sopped most of it up. We rinse out the abdomen and I start looking for the source.

I find nothing. Absolutely nothing.

I stuff the intestines back inside and suture up the midline incision. As I take off the drape, I glance at the urinary catheter and see pus coming out instead of urine.

Of course, a severe kidney infection. We've already given IV antibiotics and I write on the orders to continue them. He has been stable throughout the surgery and we move him out to the ward.

The next morning he is doing a little better but still breathing fast and not really waking up. His urine has cleared up though and his heart rate has decreased.

Half way through the day the nurses call me to see him. I rush over expecting the worst, but find that he is actually a little improved over the morning. It seems like he'll make it.

That night, the nurse calls me to see a kid she's admitting. I go over to the Pediatric ward and notice an empty bed.

The little boy died a few hours ago.

I collapse against the wall and close my eyes. I can't wait for the day when "He will wipe every tear from their eyes. There will be no more death or mourning or crying or pain, for the old order of things has passed away."

08 July 2007
Mistakes

I open Marie's belly. Marie is a woman with a large lower abdominal mass. A huge smooth, lumpy, solid but not hard, mass fills her entire pelvis. I identify the right ovary and tube with what appears to be a fibroma sticking out behind and a huge fibroma filling the rest of the belly.

I start to remove the uterus, but it's difficult because there's no room to maneuver to get down the side to the base. I do most of the right side and then move over to the left. That's where I start to make mistakes because I misdiagnosed the problem.

It's already taken an hour and a half. We're using Ketamine general anesthesia which means no muscle relaxation. The whole time I've been trying to keep all the intestines out of the already cramped pelvis. I'm moving down the uterus staying close to it like I've been trained to do to avoid the ureters when I cut through the ureter.

Mistake number two. The first one I won't discover till later.

I realize I'll have to repair the ureter later so I tag it and keep moving. Finally, I get low enough where it's time to separate the bladder from the cervix. It's stuck. As I try to free it, I enter the bladder which is weird because their doesn't seem to be really any uterus behind it.

Mistake number three.

I decide to open up the uterus and take out the fibromas to free up some space and try to identify things better. I make the incision and find thick, jelly-like contents. It's a huge mucinous ovarian cyst that has attached to the uterus making it seem like a fibroma.

I shell it out and suddenly, the normal sized, half taken out uterus appears in the right pelvis. I then look back at what I thought were the enlarged uterine vessels and realize I've probably cut the femoral vessels. I ask Siméon to feel the left leg.

He's says it's a lot colder than the right.

I'm getting desperate. In my ignorance I've probably cost this lady her leg and kidney. We're already two hours into the surgery, the leg has been without blood for 30 minutes already and I still have to take out the uterus and the rest of the ovary. Only then can I try and do something about the artery, vein, ureter and bladder.

I'm fighting off panic. I want to rush. I have to make myself calm down. Do I have what it takes?

I've been praying almost continuously that God won't make my stupidity or ignorance or whatever you call it ruin this woman's life.

While panic still lurks right under the surface, I feel somehow that I'm not alone in this. I have a mentor, an attending physician with me who says, "I'm not going to take over. I've given you what you need. I'll walk you through it."

I suture up the bladder in two layers.

I search for the femoral vein first. I find both ends of a large severed vein in the right place now that the anatomy is clear. I clamp them with vascular clamps before cutting off the sutures and trimming the ends. I find the proximal end of the artery but can't really find the distal end.

I take some very fine suture and painstakingly put in the sutures starting from the back side and working around to the front. Abel, my assistant, is fighting a never-ending battle against the intestines, the oozing blood and fluids, and the vein itself that doesn't want to stay close enough to suture.

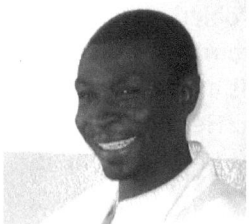

Abel

In the meantime, Siméon has done a hemoglobin. The results come back: 6.0 g/dl. He's ordered a blood transfusion.

I release the clamps and a huge clot bursts out followed by dark blood rapidly filling the operating field. We suction and mop up desperately as I reattach the clamp. I suture a bit more where it's leaking and try again.

Same thing. I'm trying hard not to get desperate and just quit. Finally, we release the clamps again and there's no bleeding.

I start the search for the distal part of the artery. I just can't seem to find it. I release the clamp I thought was holding the artery to try and attach it better. It turns out to be a branch of the vein as dark blood immediately begins to gush out. We repeat the same process until it's definitely stopped.

I hunt and hunt for the artery. It has to be here. Finally, I find and clamp it. I start the slow process of suturing with fine suture. We are four hours into the surgery, two hours without blood to the leg.

I release the clamps on the artery. There is no bleeding, but no real pulsation either. It's probably clotted up. I don't know what else to do so I head to the ureter.

I always wondered what we were going to do with all those ureteral stints that someone put in the container of supplies we got two years ago, but I'm glad for them now. I open up one of the stents, slide it into both ends of the severed ureter making sure it goes all the way into the bladder, and suture up the ureter around it.

Finally, we close up the abdomen and I check her leg.

Is it my imagination, or does she have a faint pulse in her foot? The leg is still cool. Only time will tell. We put her on some Heparin and Diclofenac, the only blood thinners we have and pray for the best.

I don't know how to explain it, but as I walk out, instead of feeling stressed and annoyed, I almost feel refreshed, even though my body is tired. It has been a time when I knew God was with me. He didn't say "Well, you caused the problem so you're on your own." Rather, He encouraged me, kept me from giving up and led me through.

Two days later, her leg is a little swollen, but she has a good pulse and can move her leg normally. Her urine is clear, her intestinal function has returned and she's starting to take oral fluids.

22 July 2007
Waste

As I enter the theater, the old Arab man is sitting upright on the table ready for his spinal anesthesia. He has two bulges sticking out of each side of his lower abdomen. He bends as far as his arthritic back will let him. Miraculously, the needle goes straight in despite his twisted, calcified spine and I inject the spinal anesthetic.

We lay him down quickly and tilt the head of the table down. Odei has already scrubbed and is putting his sterile gloves on. I scrub and join him. After draping him with the sterile towels we pause and pray as usual.

I start on the right side. It's a hernia all right but not the traditional one. Half his intestines have come through his abdominal wall through the hole where the spermatic cord comes out, but instead of going down the canal into the scrotum it has wormed it's way under the skin of the belly.

It's fairly easy to dissect out since it's not attached to the cord. I bury the sac inside with a purse string suture and close the weak area with mesh so there's no tension. I repeat the same thing on the left side. A little over an hour has passed and the patient is doing well.

Two operations down, one to go. I make a small midline incision over the distended bladder and enter the bladder easily. Urine gushes out. I suction rapidly and ask them to unclamp the foley catheter. Nothing comes out below but urine continues to pour out from above. When I've finally sucked up all the urine I ask Abel if it was difficult to get the foley in. He says, yes, he had to force it.

Great. I look in the bladder. I see the bulging prostate but there's no catheter. I stick my finger into the middle of the prostate and start scooping it out in a circular motion starting at the left around to the back and then to the right. It comes out cleanly and easily.

I then ask Siméon to reinsert the large bore three way foley. It won't enter the bladder. I feel down in the mush of blood clots that used to house the prostate and I can't feel the urethral opening for anything.

Either Abel's created a false track that the foley prefers to the real one or the man also has a urethral stricture. We try and try to insert the catheter as the blood continues to well out of the bladder. Nothing.

We try passing a urethral dilator. Nothing. I try passing one from above but still can't find the urethral opening. I'm not sure how much time passes, but it seems like forever.

Finally, I'm able to find the urethra with a dilator and it comes out the penis. I then have Siméon attach a large suture which I pull back into the bladder and detach from the dilator. Siméon then threads the suture through the opening in the foley and inserts it while I pull from above. Finally, the catheter enters the bladder.

By this time, the spinal has worn off and we have to give him Ketamine. He starts to react by contracting all his muscles making it impossible to continue the operation. Finally, with Diazepam and Chlorpromazine, he relaxes.

I close up the bladder in two layers, the balloon on the foley is blown up and pulled into the prostatic fossa, and irrigation of the bladder is started. I close the fascia and skin and take off the gown.

I look at the monitor: blood pressure is normal, pulse is a little elevated but not much considering the effect of Ketamine and surgery, oxygen saturation is normal, he is breathing easily on his own.

A half an hour later a nurse comes running. "James, come quick, the patient's not breathing."

I run over to the surgical ward where I find a crowd of Arabs around a cold body with no pulse or respiratory effort. I am about to give my condolences and walk away but something pushes me in the opposite direction.

"Bring the gurney," I shout as I start chest compressions. The nurses arrive quickly, but not before my vigorous CPR has led to a few cracked ribs. I continue the compressions as we race to the operating room.

In the operating room, Abel takes over compressions as I whip out the intubation kit and place an endotracheal tube. Odei does CPR while Abel attaches the cardiac monitor.

Flatline, Oxygen sat 28%, no pulse. We continue. Electrical activity starts to come and go on the monitor. We try adrenaline and atropine.

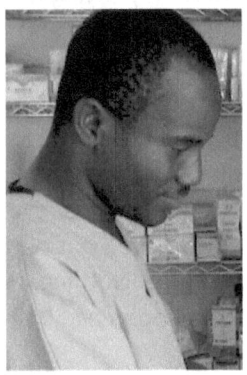

Odei

There seems to be electrical activity but the rate is slow. Still no pulse. Abel and Odei haven't done much CPR, but with my encouragement they are really pumping vigorously as I squeeze the bag to breath for the patient since we have no ventilator.

Suddenly, there is good electrical activity. I ask them to stop the chest compressions, sure enough, there's a booming carotid pulse. His O2 sat is up to 90%. We keep bagging. I add some IV glucose. Abel makes sure the bladder irrigation isn't blocked.

Still no neurologic response.

I notice his blood pressure is hanging on the very low end of normal. As Sarah takes over bagging I start to leaf through an anesthesia book. Look, a chapter on the elderly. Interesting, their adrenal function is diminished. I look up onto the anesthesia cart and my eyes light on the hydrocortisone. I'd secretly wondered why the Romanian orthopedists had brought and left it for us.

I quickly give our Arab man 100mg and, shockingly, five minutes later his blood pressure is up to normal.

We had brought him to the operating room as he was on his Arabic rug with his prayer shawl, little skull cap and two sets of Muslim prayer beads. He is covered with a piece of cloth with a picture of Jesus on it surrounded by the words *Je suis le Chemin, la Verite et la Vie* (I am the Way, the Truth and the Life).

The family wants to know what's going on. We've been inside with the patient for three hours now. I invite the brother in and tell him that his sibling has been resurrected by the power of *Isa Al-Masih* who is the way the truth and the LIFE.

"Al hamdullilah" the brother states with a smile as he is escorted out.

30 minutes later, the man has started to breath on his own. I pull out his breathing tube and leave him on the oxygen concentrator for several minutes. I slowly turn the oxygen down. He continues to breath spontaneously. I turn the oxygen off. I watch him for 15 minutes and he breathes fine with a normal O2 sat. He's still not awake though. Since we don't have oxygen tanks, an ICU or ventilators, we are forced to finally just take the risk and send him back to the ward.

I call in all the family members. Over 20 robed Arab men and veiled Arab women crowd around. I explain how to keep his airway open and to how to watch his breathing and how to notify the nurse. Then I explain that they've all witnessed a miracle. He was dead, but now he's alive thanks to *Isa Al-Masih*.

I ask Odei to pray in Arabic. Wisely he turns to them with outstretched palms open towards heaven and says, *"Al Fatiha"*.

Over 20 pairs of hands come up and heads are raised as each one individually repeats his prayer of thanks to Allah. At the end, there are smiles all around with much mumbling of *"Al hamdulillah"*, *"Mashallah"* and *"Barakatullah"*.

At 3:00am, I am called to see him. He is barely breathing. We repeat the resuscitation until 7:00am. He is back alive but also has a tension pneumothorax. As I slice open the side of his chest and poke a hemostat into his lung a long hiss of pressurized air comes out. He also has anemia so we transfuse some blood. We keep him in a corner of the operating room to continue to ventilate him.

I have other cases. The first is a 10 cm ovarian cyst trapped in the broad ligament. Then, I do a hernia and take out a small lipoma.

Our Arab friend is still alive, but not breathing on his own. His face, neck and chest are swollen from subcutaneous air from the pneumothorax. We turn the breathing over to the family members.

He makes it until 2:00am the next morning until he dies.

I'm so exhausted that I can't really do my work right the next two days. I basically neglect the other hospitalized patients. Was it a waste? Did I poorly use the resource of myself? I may never know. Only God truly knows.

06 August 2007
Chronic

I only get to really know two classes of patients: ones hospitalized with chronic wounds and AIDS patients. There are really no other chronic diseases here. People don't live long enough since the life expectancy is 47 years for men and 49 years for women.

For example, our little friend, Clement, has been back with us for a couple months now. He came to us three years ago with osteomyelitis of the left tibia and has now had four surgeries to try and get his bone to heal so he can walk again. Two Romanian orthopedists were the last to operate on him in May and he's slowly but surely healing.

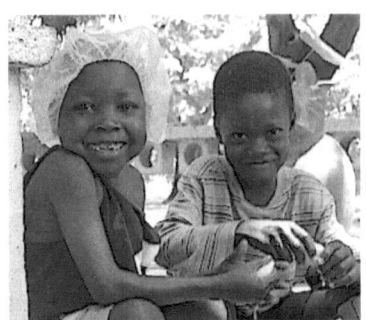

Ramadan & Clement

In the next bed over is Ramadan. He also has osteomyelitis except that his is on the right. He has been with us now for only two months. Both of them love it when we come on rounds. Their faces light up and they each try to outdo each other in slapping my hand hardest in giving me "five". Sarah also entertains them with the occasional balloon, animals drawn on their hands with markers or empty syringes she's taught them to use as water guns.

Two days ago, after giving me "five", Clement held out a handful of fresh, un-roasted peanuts insisting that I take them. Even though I know he doesn't get enough to eat, how could I refuse his generosity coming from such a pure heart?

The other patients I really get to know are our AIDS patients. I consult them for free to encourage them to come to the hospital whenever they're sick without waiting too long at home hoping it'll "just get better." We also only make them pay half price for lab tests and medications.

Once they are in full blown AIDS, we are able to treat them for free, thanks to generous donors. We give them triple anti-retroviral (ARV) therapy and all other medications as needed for opportunistic infections. Each week, when they come to get a week's supply of ARV, we have a meeting to discuss problems, teach them how to care for their health, how to recognize sickness and how to avoid transmission.

I get to know them very well. The down side, of course, is that I have to watch many of them die.

Koumabeng Chantal is an exceptional case. When I first arrived in Béré, she was already considered a "*cas social*" and was treated free by the hospital. She was eight years old, an orphan taken care of by a mentally slow, yet very loving grandma. I thought for several years that she was a "*cas social*" due to her being an orphan. It's so rare for a child given HIV by her mother during pregnancy or delivery to live past five years that I was sure she couldn't be HIV positive.

I was wrong.

Before I came, HIV was kept a secret from patients and staff. Therefore, there was no record of an HIV test done on Chantal. She was in good health overall. I treated her for several bouts of simple Malaria and some ear infections over the years. The only thing that gave me a clue that she might be immunocompromised were the umbilicated nodules on her face and arms, like tiny, fat donuts (*molluscum contagiosum*). But I'd found them on other children here who tested negative, so I didn't think much of it.

When I came back from furlough this year, Chantal came to see me and I noticed she was getting quite thin. She had another ear infection and malaria again. This time, I decided to test her for HIV. She came pack positive. I was shocked. She was now 11 years old. How had she lived so long?

I started her on ARVs which she tolerated well. She was faithful in taking them I thought. At least, she came back each week to get her next week's supply. Two months ago, she came in with a severe headache. She was in such pain that she cried and moaned all night long keeping all the other patients awake. I was afraid of some opportunistic infection like Toxoplasmosis, but she did have severe malaria so I decided to treat her for that first before thinking of something else.

After three days, she went home pain free to finish her malaria treatment at home. A month later, she repeated the same thing. She was suffering horribly. This time she needed five days of IV Quinine before the malaria and headache cleared.

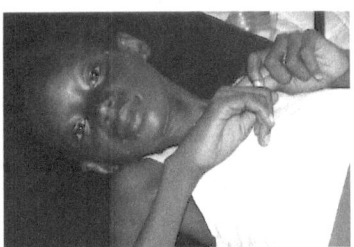

Chantal

Now, she's in my office again. As always she is gentle and subdued with big trusting eyes. As I gaze into that unblinking stare I see the quiet suffering. She only whimpers as I lay her on the exam table. Her only complaint is headache and vomiting.

Her malaria smear comes back very positive at 0,20%. We hospitalize her again and try a new, once-a-day anti-malarial called Artemether. A single shot in the thigh once a day without all the side effects of Quinine.

Every day, I go to see her. She lies there quietly, her form thin, but not emaciated and that same look in her eyes. One eye is slightly crosseyed. Her grandma says she refuses to eat and has vomited several times. I decide to put her back on IV Quinine. Her vital signs are stable and with some Tylenol and Ibuprofen, she doesn't have hardly any pain.

That night, the nurse goes to place her evening perfusion. She calmly looks up at him and tells him it's not necessary, she's going to die. He reassures her that things will be fine even though she's not afraid and seems completely at peace. He starts the drip and moves on as she falls into a deep sleep.

At 2:00am, she quietly stops breathing. She's gone.

14 August 2007
Baby Hernia

Friday. The end of a long week. I'm set to travel Sunday to N'Djamena. The day is almost over. It's been pretty quiet.

"Docteur, you should see this case." Jacob pokes his head in my office at around noon.

A tall, lean father with his young wife wrapped in a bright blue and yellow patterned body wrap walks in carrying a chubby little three month old. He's sleeping quietly. The mom sits on the exam table and unwraps the baby exposing the obvious problem.

His left groin and scrotum is swollen to 10 times the normal size. I palpate it and with gentle pressure the "mass" slithers back into the belly causing the child to wake up and cry. My finger is in a hole in the inguinal canal. When I release, the cries cause the baby's intestines to pop right back out.

If I wait, the intestines could get trapped outside. Since I'm leaving Sunday, I should operate today even though I'm tired. Samedi, Abel and Siméon all try tirelessly to find an IV without success. Finally, we are forced to use intramuscular Ketamine for the anesthesia.

Abel straps the tiny infant onto a "papoose board" so he can't move while Siméon applies Betadine generously to his abdomen, groin, scrotum, penis and upper legs. I open the hernia pack, scrub, pull on sterile gown and gloves and pick up the scalpel. It seems so big compared to the little body now draped in sterile towels.

I gently slice a two centimeter incision over the still bulging hernia. The sac is so thin I can see the intestines inside. It reaches all the way down to the testicle. It is a delicate thing to dissect off the spermatic cord from the thin sac and it tears in a couple places but finally is free.

I push in the intestines and clamp off the sac. I tie it closed and cut off the rest of the sac. This is where I briefly think of doing something I regret not doing later. Everything I've just read says that tying off the sac in infants is almost always enough with just a 1% chance of recurrence. So, I decide not to close the hernia defect but just close the fascia over the spermatic cord. I attach the testicle to the scrotum with a button on the outside and close up the skin. He did well under anesthesia and I go home.

The next day is Saturday. I don't do rounds until the afternoon. I come up to see the nurse and he says that I need to see the baby I operated on yesterday, his scrotum is swollen up. I have a sinking feeling in my stomach as I walk down the dimly lit corridor to the bare bones hospital ward packed with visitors.

The baby looks sick. He is somewhat lethargic and has a rapid heartbeat and is a little pale. His scrotum is swollen and edematous. It's not readily obvious if it's the hernia come back or a hematoma. I ask the father and he says the swelling started on the inferior part of the scrotum and worked it's way up.

Looks like a hematoma, but I'm not sure. I feel a sense of helplessness. If it's the hernia he'll die without an operation, but he's so sick he won't survive another operation. And I'm leaving tomorrow morning early.

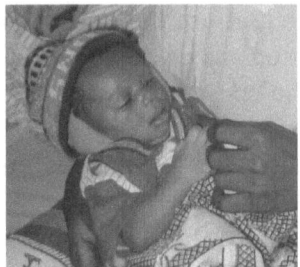

Hernia baby

I make a tough decision to not operate. I suspect he has malaria as well, so I treat his malaria and hope it's just a hematoma that will resolve itself. I don't feel good about my decision, but go home with a heavy heart. I'm sure I'll never see him again.

The next day is an early day. I get on a *moto-taxi* and as I pull away from the hospital I can't help but wondering if the baby's not already dead.

I get back to Béré at midnight Wednesday after getting stuck in the mud right before the barge crossing, just a few kilometers from Béré. By the time I eat and hit the sack it's 1:30am. I sleep till almost 10:00am the next morning before going up to the hospital.

To my surprise, the baby is still alive and looking a lot better. He is alert and bright eyed, but his belly is very swollen and he's still pale. He now has an IV that has given him some much needed IV fluids. I check his hemoglobin which is barely over 6.0 g/dl, about a third of normal. I order a blood transfusion.

The scrotum is still swollen and it's obvious now that it's the hernia that's come back. I take him to surgery as the blood transfusion runs in. Odei assists me as I incise larger and perpendicular to the old incision. A mass of swollen, dark red intestines pop into the field. I try to push them back in but without muscle relaxation and an already swollen abdomen, it's all but impossible.

It seems like the intestine is still viable. I push and push but can't get it all inside. It starts to get darker. The blood supply is being cut off before my very eyes. I'm feeling desperate and am sweating and swearing under my breath. Then, part of the intestine tears partway through. Thankfully, the inner part doesn't tear but now I have to take out part of the intestine. I open the appropriate instrument pack, put bowel clamps over where the intestine looks nice and pink. Then I clamp off the blood vessels supplying the dying part and cut it out.

Now, I'm stuck trying to suture the tiniest of small intestines in a field only about 3cm big. I make a ton of tiny interrupted stitches through the inner lining and then run a second layer through the tougher muscle layer. I release the bowel clamps. Air and stool inflates the newly sewn intestine without leakage. I'm able to push the rest of the intestine inside. I take out the testicle and cut and tie the cord pushing the stump inside. Then I close the fascia and all the the rest in three layers.

I close my cross shaped incision. The kid's still alive though his belly is tense and he's not breathing that well. I put him on IV fluids and antibiotics and tell his parents to not let him breastfeed or take anything to drink.

He's still alive the next few days but his belly is still very swollen.

Three days later, I come in to the hospital for rounds and the baby's belly is flat and soft. He's been farting and pooping. His vital signs are normal. The wound is healing well and he's breast-feeding. He pulls away from the breast and looks up at me with clear eyes.

16 August 2007

Marie

I'm poised over Marie's body, scalpel in hand. It's hard to believe that this will be the third major surgery on this poor woman in a month. I've been torn inside as to whether this is the right thing to do, but now as I stand ready to cut, I feel peace.

"Let's pray."

As Samedi prays in Nangjéré I find images rapidly running through my mind: Huge mass. Cut ureter. Tied femoral vessels. Realizing what I've done. Meticulous suturing. Four hour surgery. Feeling of failure. Swollen leg. Alive. Slow but sure recovery. Discharge. Return a week later with swollen belly. Ultrasound showing loculated fluid. Is it tumor or leaking urine? Abdominal surgery again. Belly full of yellow liquid. Every surface inflamed and stuck together. Jelly like substance on everything. Retention sutures. Two drains. Three weeks in the hospital with liters of fluid still coming out. Uncertainty. If it's the leaking ureter I should take out her kidney. If it's the tumor, why put her through another major operation. Today, there's pus coming out the drain. I can't wait longer.

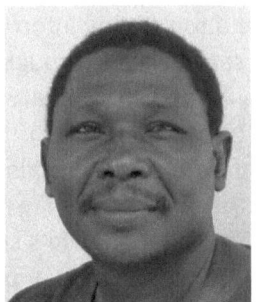

Samedi

When Samedi finishes his prayer, I open my eyes and slice from the bottom of her last rib, across her side to in front of her pelvic bone. I use the electric cautery to slowly go through fat, fascia and the different muscle layers. I open the cavity over the kidney. I dissect out the fat. I slowly release the fine fibers attaching the kidney surface to the surrounding tissues. I work my way deep in and around the top part taking off the adrenal gland. Then around the bottom part and the back. Finally I find the huge renal artery and vein. I delicately strip off the fat till I can see it well. It's so deep. I'm trying to not shake in my nervousness. If I don't tie it off well, she could bleed out quickly. I don't really have the right instruments. I finally get three clamps on the artery. I cut the artery and tie the part I'm leaving in two places and the part I'm taking out in one. The vein is huge and branches right under where I've cut the artery. I have to go deeper. Finally I clamp it and cut it. Then the ureter is clamped and cut. I pull out the kidney and tie off the ureteral stump. Then I tie off the vein twice and release the clamp. Blood surges into the field. I clamp the stump quickly, put it under a little tension while Samedi suctions till I can see where it's bleeding and clamp that. I tie it off. I release it. No bleeding. I close.

Marie goes home a week later completely healed. I know that what I have done I am incapable of having done. But that's the cool thing about working here, God puts me in situations where I know I can't do it, and then when I do, I can't help but give him the credit.

19 August 2007
How To Catch a Wife

I follow the shadows of Samedi and Abré in front of me. With just stars to light the way, we head to Abré's house winding among the shadows in the shapes of pointed roofed huts, trees, tall millet stalks and brick fences.

We round a corner and the shadows dance on the walls of the compound in the flickering light of a kerosene lamp as the shadow of Abré's wife brings in some wooden stools for us to sit on. Then she returns for the formal greeting of curtsying at the waist and bending the knees to present her hand bent at a 45 degree angle down to be shaken by each visitor.

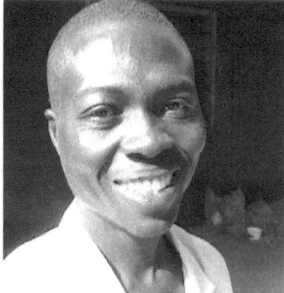

Abré

Abré presents his problem. He's asked Samedi and I to come give him advice. Once the advice has been adequately discussed and accepted, Abré's wife brings out a small metal pot filled with pasta shells and a goat meat sauce. The meal is set on the rickety wooden coffee table. We lean forward and dig in with our large, flimsy spoons.

As we sit up, bellies full, I ask Abré what I think will be a simple question. It turns out to be a long, twisted story that I don't really understand until later.

"Abré, how did you meet your wife?"

Abré clears his throat and starts spinning his tale in his rich, deep baritone voice.

"I was back in my village, Kalmé. I'd come to Béré for high school. I went home on weekends. When classes were over I went home to work my field. I saw this girl from a long way off. She pleased me.

"A few days later, she came to draw water at our well. I had a mango in my hand. I offered it to her. She didn't want it. I insisted. I asked her why I would give her a bad mango? She took it.

"When she came back to draw water a few days later, I had a bunch of mangoes to give her. We started to talk.

"I told my father that was the girl I wanted to marry. She was from a village six kilometers away but had come to go to the school in my village and was the servant of my neighbor.

"My dad said it wasn't wise to get a girl from that village, but it was up to me. He would pay the dowry, but then it was up to me. So he did.

"Half-way through the next school year, I decided it was time to find her. I heard she was in a certain village. I went there with my friends, but she had just left. I heard she was at the market, I went there with my friends, but she wasn't there. Finally, I heard she was back in Kalmé. I went there to the house where she'd been a servant. She wasn't there.

"I knew then she was back at her parents' house. I called together three of my strongest friends. I told them that tonight was the night. They nodded and we left at 10:00pm to walk to the girl's village. When we got to the outskirts, I told my friends to wait. I left my bike a little farther on under a certain tree.

"I snuck into the village and stole into the girl's family compound. Stealthily, I made my way to her hut. I knocked on the door. No answer. I knocked again. Still nothing. I knocked again and whispered loudly 'it's me.' She opened the door and told me to leave. I refused. I told her to come out and go get my bike under such and such a tree. She said no so I grabbed her hand and made her come with me. She fought, but not loudly enough to wake her family.

"I brought her to my bike and then to my friends. We took her by force home to my village that very night. We got in at 5:00am. That's how I got my wife."

I'm sitting there stunned. Not exactly the romantic love story I'd hoped for. Fortunately, before I can say anything stupid, Samedi pipes up with an explanation.

"That's our tradition. The woman should be stolen from her family by the man who's paid the dowry. He should get his strongest friends to go with him because the family will resist and if he's not strong enough to take his wife be force they'll beat him up. Then, a week later, the girl will get her girlfriend's together and they'll go to the boy for the marriage. But everyone will make fun of him and say he wasn't strong enough to fight for his woman. So, you need to strategize, come at night and bring some tough guys with you if you want to be respected."

The next night, I'm sitting around a similar table with our Pastor Dieudonné Atchouma. The only difference is this time the area is well lit. I tell him the story Abré told me last night.

"That's nothing," he said. "You should check out the tribe around Bongor. Their women are tough. They all know how to use a bow staff like the Chinese. From an early age, the girls practice out in the fields. When you want to get married, after you pay the dowry, you are sent off into the bush with the woman and you have to fight her. If you can't beat her, she'll pound you to a pulp and send you home with your tail between your legs and you'll have to find another woman. If you beat her, however, and are able to disarm, capture, and bring her home, then you've earned the village's respect and you can marry her.

"Those women are fierce. Back in the days of the German colonists, they tried to conquer this people. They had guns and everything but they were beaten back by the women with their bow staffs. They're hard-core."

03 September 2007
Dabegue

The pouring down rain soaks through my jeans and fogs up my glasses. Sarah and I have saddled up the horses, packed medicines in the saddlebags and are on our way to Noel's.

The two meter tall millet and corn leans out haphazardly over the winding, mud puddle filled road across the Western edge of Béré. I get slapped in the face and chest several times with the long, firm heads on the weaving stalks as the horse gallops back and forth in the slalom course of small ponds, dodging ducks and frogs along the way.

Noel's house is the last one on the road that heads to Delbian, Bao and Moundou. It's a conglomerate of partially finished mud brick buildings. Some are without roof, doors and windows. Some have tin used for all of the above. He is waiting outside leaning his chair back against the wall.

Noel was trained by the Russians and Libyans to be a terrorist, but found God in a refugee camp in West Africa. He is now our hospital chaplain is dressed in a maroon robe with a black and red striped Arab hat sitting on his shaved head. He sports a scruffy goatee and partial beard already tinged with gray.

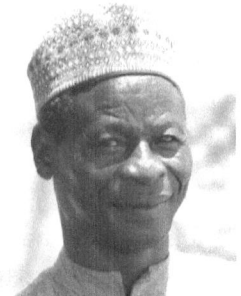

Noel

He manages to get on the third horse after a couple of attempts and we're off to Dabegue.

After a couple kilometers we enter the village which stretches for about five kilometers, hugging the road without much depth. It's just a rough collection of mud hut compounds interspersed with fields of rice, millet, corn, peanuts and sweet potatoes.

Halfway through the village we turn at what's left of a burned out tree trunk that was struck by lightening years ago. We weave through a narrow passage with millet stalks swaying on both sides and come out in the open under a large mango tree with a mud brick wall on the left. Two rickety wooden chairs made low to the ground and leaned back for lounging are gathered around a rickety metal coffee table.

Our host hurries out to greet us with his wife. They both look familiar. I don't figure out how I know them till a little later. All I can say is I'm amazed at how God can work even through our mistakes.

It doesn't take long for kids to pour in from all directions. They take their places on a large mat with four galloping horses woven into the pattern in yellow and red. Noel pulls out two Bible picture rolls. At first the kids are shy with two strangers there. Noel tries to teach them a song in Nangjéré but no one gets into it until we make it a competition. Noel and the guys sing against me and the girls to see who can make the most noise!

Noel then calls up the kids to say what they can name from the picture story of last week. They are so proud to recognize Mary, Joseph, Jesus and the wise men, getting a round of applause led by Noel each time.

The toothy grins and laughter are contagious. I'm having a great time trying to pick up some Nangjéré here and there as Noel continues the story of Jesus.

After 15 minutes we sing another song and then I get to try and answer the adults' questions from last week. The first question is why horses and lions don't get along these days like they do in the picture of Adam in the Garden of Eden.

I talk in French and Noel translates into Nangjéré. They all understand about the serpent (Genesis 3) and how it is really the devil who made war against God by rebelling against him (Revelation 12) and how it came about through his pride and ambition to be like God (Isaiah 14 and Ezekiel 28). It seems to make sense that after the flood when God tells Noah that he'll make the animals afraid of humans (Genesis 9) that it's the result of rebellion why horses and lions just don't get along.

We finish after about 30 minutes. Sarah and I then start to consult some sick kids. We've brought a battery powered device to check hemoglobins and find five kids with severe anemia (hemoglobin of 5.0 g/dl or less) due to malaria. We refer them to the hospital for blood transfusions. The rest we treat for Malaria and parasites. We see 80 kids in a little over an hour.

After a meal of boiled eggs, steamed corn, chicken and rice we pack up to go home.

Half an hour after arriving home, Tchibtchang knocks on the door. Tall and stern, Tchibtchang is one of our newest and best nurses. Dressed in bright aqua scrubs and a long white coat I know he must have a case for me.

He starts to talk about several patients, but I quickly realize I need to see them in person so I walk over to the hospital with him.

We head first to labor and delivery. The room is dark and there is a young woman, obviously pregnant stretched out on her left side on the exam table. It's her first pregnancy and she's been in our hospital in labor since 3:00am today. She has been fully dilated for hours and can't deliver.

I have her turn onto her back and grab the fetal doppler off the table. I squirt a glob of ultrasound jelly onto her belly between her belly button and her right pelvis. I stretch out the doppler stick on its telephone-like cord to place it on the jelly. I fire up the device to a reassuring crackle as the move it gently over the belly. In the right lower quadrant I hear the reassuring boom-boom, boom-boom of a rapid fetal heart beat running at 140 per minute.

The baby's still alive.

I hurry to the operating room and get the symphysiotomy kit, a suture, a scalpel, a razor blade, some gauze sponges, Betadine, a syringe, some lidocaine, a foley catheter with bag, a pair of sterile gloves and a vacuum extractor.

While Tchibtchang inserts the urinary catheter I shave the pubic area with the razor, prep it with Betadine and inject 10mL of lidocaine into the skin then around and in the cartilage of the pubis.

I open the symphysiotomy kit, attach a large scalpel to the scalpel holder and make a small incision all the way down to the cartilage. I then stick my other hand inside to move the urinary catheter to the side effectively displacing the urethra. I slice through the cartilage which cuts remarkably easily until I'm most of the way through.

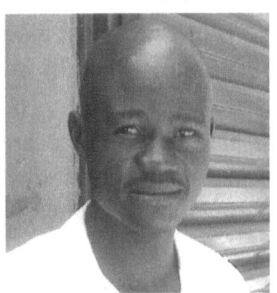

Tchibtchang

Then, Tchibtchang and Odei pull the legs up, out and down until we hear a pop and feel the pelvis come apart a few centimeters. She has a contraction. I attach the vacuum pump to the fetal head. I make an lateral episiotomy with the surgical scissors to open up the vaginal opening and with one push the baby is out.

His face wrinkles up and his arms and legs are nicely flexed but he doesn't cry or breath. I suck out the green, meconium thick fluid out of his mouth and nose, clamp the umbilical cord, cut between the clamps and take him over to the resuscitation table.

He has a good heart beat but still doesn't want to breath. I rough him up a little on his spine and feet while vigorously drying him off.

Still no cry.

I pump his chest a little and put a tiny mask on his face and give him a few breaths.

Finally he lets out a little whimper. I continue my shaking and rubbing and he finally starts to breath and wail.

I return to the mom, pull out the placenta, suture up the symphysiotomy wound in two layers and then repair the episiotomy.

Tchibtchang then takes me to see the next two cases.

The first is a four year old girl with fever and abdominal pain. They've started her on a quinine drip. I look at her, and I can't explain why, but I feel there's something else going on. There's no vomiting, but hasn't pooped in two days. She doesn't really want to eat, but has taken some porridge. Her eyes look kind of glazed over. The abdominal pain could be just malaria or constipation.

I feel her belly. It's soft but tender. She kind of whimpers when I touch her but it doesn't seem too bad.

For some reason, something bothers me, though. I decide to do a rectal exam. She seems tender on the right and not the left.

I'm afraid it might be appendicitis, but I'm nervous about operating. She'd come in the morning with anemia and had been transfused. Maybe it's just severe malaria. If it is, I could kill her by operating.

I decide to buy some time. I order antibiotics and more IV fluids while I go look at the next patient.

This one is straight forward, a strangulated hernia. The hernia is massive, painful and won't go back inside. He's vomited once.

We take him straight to the operating room.

I make a large diagonal incision directly over the bulging hernia. I dissect the sack free from the spermatic cord and the contents pop back in to the abdomen. I take out the testicle, tie off the sack and stitch a piece of sterilized mosquito netting over the week spot between the transversalis fascia and the inguinal ligament. He's 60 years old and doesn't need more than one testicle anyway and this way it's sure not to recur. I close up the fascia and skin, take off my gloves and go back to see the four year old girl.

Something still bothers me and I make a tough decision. I tell the father that she'll die without an operation but she might die during the surgery. Does he want us to go through with it? He's agrees, so we wheel her off to the operating room.

Siméon gives her Ketamine. Abel preps the belly with Betadine and drapes it with sterile towels. I use the tubal ligation kit which has smaller retractors for this tiny abdomen.

I pray as usual and then slice carefully through the thin skin, tiny fascia and muscles. I gently enter the peritoneal cavity.

Purulent fluid and dark bowels bulge out letting me know instantly it was a good decision to operate. I enlarge the abdominal wound and out pops a blackened small intestine, so necrotic it's at the point of perforating but appears to have held itself intact so far.

I break away some adhesions and free up the bowel. The black, dusky parts go almost all the way to the large intestine on the distal end and about a foot and a half proximally.

I open the laparotomy kit and pull out the bowel clamps. I put one clamp over healthy intestine and then a second one over the part to be removed. I then clamp off the vessels feeding the dead intestine and remove it all together.

I tie off the vessels in the mesentery and then examine the two ends of remaining intestine. the proximal end looks good but the distal end looks dead. I'm worried because there's only about 2-3 cm of intestine left until the colon. It'll be much more difficult if I have to open the colon to reattach the small intestine. I remove one centimeter more leaving just barely over a centimeter that now looks fairly healthy.

I suture the tiny small bowel with tiny sutures and then do a second layer. I take off the clamps and there is no leaking or bleeding. I insert two drains.

Then she starts to vomit. And vomit. And vomit. Dark green with black coffee grounds. We insert an nasogastric tube and get almost half a liter out of her stomach. I wash out the abdomen with a lot of fluids, close the fascia and skin, and place a bandage.

I prescribe antibiotics and IV fluids. I tell the family not to give her anything to eat or drink. I go home.

The next day, the woman and her baby, the man with the hernia and the little girl are all still alive.

Al hamdullilah!

19 September 2007

Dragonflies

I live in a world of incredible suffering and stunning beauty.

Nasara Encore

As the tall grass itches the backs of my calves I let myself down to the ground. I slip off my white and orange Crocs and use them as a mat. The soccer match is already underway.

The agility, grace and power of the players makes me forget their ages until halftime. Sporting white t-shirts with their names hand painted on the back, the team rushes by me yelling my name and shouting *lapia*. It's then I remember they're just little kids.

They come back skipping, laughing and smiling, each with a half-eaten, half-ripe guava in hand ready for the second half.

There is not a single artificial sound to be heard, just the gentle rustle of the breeze in the drying out remnants of the millet harvest, the distant shouts and babble of the kids joking in Nangjéré and the buzz of a million dragonfly wings.

I let my focus drift from the sprawling lushness of the rainy season transforming the African bush and onto a sky so startlingly blue it almost hurts to the hundreds of seeming motionless hovering dragonflies. They are evenly spaced about a meter apart and at seemingly haphazard levels that nonetheless give a sense of order in some weird mathematical way.

The light has taken on that quality one only finds right before the sun sets low enough to turn color. The billowing white clouds make a perfect canvas to reflect the brilliance of the sun's perfect angle and to mute it so it brings out everything in detailed sharpness.

I feel transported to another time and another place. A time and a place where I'm not watching babies die every day. A time and a place where it's almost unheard of for a woman to have lost a child tragically. A time and a place where I'm not the only doctor for hundreds of thousands of the poor and oppressed. A time and a place where I don't feel overwhelmed almost constantly. A time and a place that for me is a fading memory reawakened occasionally by miraculous, dragonfly filled moments.

As the kids resume their match, some older boys start a small circle of soccer "foreplay". Each one takes the ball and bounces it off a knee, or feet several times, maybe a head bump or two and then passes it to the next guy, hopefully without ever letting the ball touch the ground.

Four younger kids are alternately sprawling around, running back and forth chasing a tiny, pink, half-deflated ball.

All the children on and off the field are barefoot except for one who looks like he's wearing army boots and socks three sizes to big. The score is one to one.

Behind me, I notice a newcomer on the scene: a boy about 12 or 13 years old. He's crippled. He has a single homemade wooden crutch. One leg is severely shortened causing his whole body to swerve and lean. Somehow, he still manages to join the boys in their game, kicking the ball around with both feet as he hops around on his crutch.

I call to Tabegue, Samedi's nephew and tell him I want to talk to the handicapped kid.

His story is tragic, yet all to common here in Tchad.

In 2002, he was just running and then felt his leg "give way". According to him, it was "out of joint". He had many traditional bone setters try and put it in, but it never healed right and he's been crippled ever since.

I have him lie on the ground as all the kids not playing in the match gather quickly around to watch. His left knee is about 10 inches shorter than his right. His left lower leg is normal. His hip has a surprising range of motion, but there is a bony mass sticking up, out and back.

What probably happened is something that in the developed world would be operated on right away. With the placement of a few pins, six weeks later he'd be back walking not knowing that if he'd been born in a different country, he'd be handicapped for life.

I tell him to come see me the next day at the hospital. I hope to be able to help him.

He never shows up, but the dragonflies continue to hover.

23 September 2007
Why Bother?

Sometimes I wonder why I even bother. I stand in the semidarkness of the early evening with my hand over the heart of an 11 year old girl feeling the life ebb out of her. I've detached the Ambu bag from the tracheostomy tube in her neck. She's not breathing. Her pupils are fixed and dilated. I'm now getting to experience for the first time in a raw way the process of life leaving a broken body.

She came in four days ago. She was by the side of the road drawing water from the lake that has now all but flooded the road in between Béré and Kélo. A truck was trying to plow and rev it's way through the water logged mud and slid over towards the girl. She was knocked over and the truck turned on it's side crushing her legs beneath. The passengers frantically unloaded the barrels off the truck and were able to lift the truck up enough to pull her mangled body out from under it.

She arrives at the hospital conscious with her right leg twisted out at an impossible angle and her left leg wrapped in a bloody, mud-splotched t-shirt. She has no other apparent injuries, just her two legs.

I unwrap the shirt.

Her left lower leg is sliced open from just below the knee to just above the ankle as with a butcher knife. There is another 6 inch long cut on the side, a two inch long cut on the back of the calf and an inch long wound over her outside ankle.

The large lower leg bone is broken and the pieces sticking out at weird angles with much of the rest of the bone exposed.

Her right femur is also fractured, but not open.

We start an IV, give antibiotics and put her under anesthesia. We scrub out the wounds and rinse with liters and liters of antimicrobial fluids. I set the bones which have cracked in a V-shape making the reduction fairly stable. Our new nurse volunteer, Liz holds the reduction at the foot and I suture the wounds closed.

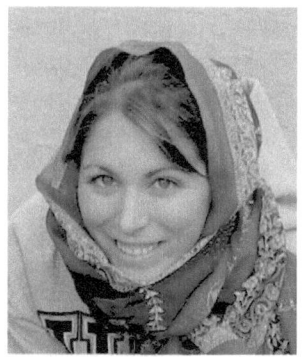

Liz

I put casts around her ankle and knee with a broken broom stick on each side to act as an external fixator. The fracture is stabilized and we have room to clean and dress the wounds.

I then drill a pin through the distal femur on her other leg. We move her to her hospital bed where I attache a sand-filled shirt to the pin with a rope to act as traction for the femur fracture.

She is breathing well and is otherwise stable.

A few hours later I go to check on her and she is in respiratory distress. She has what is every anesthesiologist's worst nightmare: micrognathia. In other words, her lower jaw never developed well and is so tiny that her mouth won't really open, her tongue is too big for her throat and her airway is small.

She has too many secretions and now her neck has started to swell. She probably had head trauma as well. She is struggling to breath sucking desperately with her chest. I run and get the pulse oximeter and her oxygen is already going down. I yell for the family members to grab her bed and carry it to the operating room since it has no wheels.

I run ahead to open up the OR. I go back and find they haven't moved. I notice she has stopped breathing. I yell again and this time they come running. We somehow manage to get the bed out of the ward, across the courtyard and into the operating room.

No breathing, no pulse.

I grab a scalpel and slice her throat. I poke aside the muscles with a clamp and expose her trachea. I cut into it with a scalpel and widen the hole with the clamp and grasp each side with hemostats. I insert an endotracheal tube into the hole and attach an Ambu bag while Anatole starts chest compressions.

Miraculously, she comes back to life. After a few minutes she is breathing on her own through the tube in her neck and after waiting a while to make sure she's stable we take her back to the ward.

She stays in a coma, however, and we realize she has brain swelling from the accident. For two days we keep the swelling down enough with medicines that she breathes on her own. Her pupils still react normally. On the third day, we have to start breathing for her. The family members take turns "bagging" her to force air into her lungs.

By the fourth day—today—the pupils are fixed and dilated.

I'm amazed at how long it can take to try and save a life and how quickly one can remove those life saving devices. Surgery took two hours. The tracheostomy and resuscitation took another hour. Not to mention all the other time spent adjusting meds, explaining to family members, suctioning her tracheostomy tube.

Now in 10 minutes her IV is out, the urinary catheter has been removed, the tracheostomy was pulled, the traction pin drilled out, and the cast cut off. Nothing remains but the sutures and the slightly twisted, un-stabilized legs.

I'm sobbing deep down but no tears come. How much have I prayed for this girl over the last four days? How much of my own time, strength and energy have I put into her despite having Malaria myself? Why do I bother?

Why does God seem to never intervene? Why does it seem I'm on my own in this?

I need to make sense of it or I'll lose my faith. My thoughts start to go crazy.

Maybe it's not God's fault at all, maybe it's ours. Maybe if this girl had a clean well or running water she wouldn't have been forced to draw from the side of the road. Maybe if the road had been paved with appropriate bridges and drainage systems the truck wouldn't have slid into her. Maybe if the hospital had better lab facilities we could've intervened to prevent any of the number of things that could be unknown contributing factors to her death.

Maybe we in the West can't go out to buy the latest Energy drink or expensive gourmet coffee without using up the resources that could have gone to furnishing clean water sources in the Third World.

Maybe we can't buy bigger and fancier gas-guzzling SUVs without wasting the money that could've gone to provide simple improved infrastructure in developing nations.

Maybe we can't spend millions of dollars on boob jobs and face lifts and liposuction without depriving bush hospitals of basic laboratory and x-ray equipment.

Maybe we can't live our comfortable lives and sit back and expect God to do the work that he has given us adequate resources, abilities, talents and time to do ourselves. Maybe God's saying, "I haven't refused to save that girl's life...

"You have."

20 October 2007
Airborne

The Land Cruiser crashes through the six foot high millet over a winding, bumpy trail towards the airstrip.

It's a cool Tchadian morning just after 6:00am.

Rich has picked up Dr. Bond, Sarah and I from the hospital and brought us out here with the pilot from Adventist Medical Aviation, Gary Roberts. Gary has recently moved here from Cameroon with his wife, Wendy, and their children, Kaleb and Cherise. We finally burst on to the airstrip. A tinge of pink lines the wisps of clouds barely clinging to the night before being swept away by the new day.

The plane looks tiny against the backdrop of grassy airstrip hacked from the African bush. Using well placed whacks with long switches a few kids guide some scattered goats across the the middle of the airstrip.

Our single prop, four-seater plane is about to go international.

Bond is a little nervous and plies Gary with all kinds of questions about flight hours, how many accidents, how much fuel the plane carries, is he going to check if there's water in the fuel. As Gary takes off the tarps and I help him detach the tie downs Bond is trying to visually inspect the plane from top to bottom. Dressed in his sport coat and sporting wild black hair streaked with gray and the beginnings of a bushy mustache, Bond looks like a Sikh version of Albert Schweitzer.

Finally, luggage weighed and packed, we squeeze ourselves in the fuselage and strap ourselves in. The engine fires up blowing in a burst of cold air through the open windows. Last minute checks in place, the windows close and Gary turns the plane around away from the sunrise. Gary then reopens a window. He yells to the night watchmen to run ahead and pull the sticks serving as goal posts out of middle of the airstrip where some kids have made a soccer field.

When all is clear, Gary pulls the throttle and we lurch forward. The plane quickly pick up speed as we bump and bounce across the airstrip. In no time we are airborne as Béré drops out from below us. We take a sharp turn over the trees to buzz the hospital.

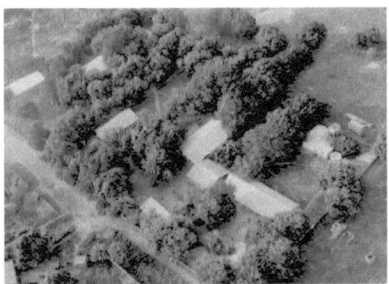

Béré Adventist Hospital

It's amazing to see how really small our 20,000 strong village really is. It's just a bunch of mud huts so well camouflaged by the mango trees and millet patches that you can hardly see anything. The only thing that really stands out are the tin roofs of the church, school and hospital as they come into view.

Seeing that tiny clump of trees with a few tin roofs jutting up it's hard to believe that anyone would want to be treated there. But people come from as far away as Lake Tchad and Abeche on the border of Darfur to be operated on in our collection of ragged buildings.

Soon we are crossing a patchwork quilt of rice, millet, peanut and sweet potato fields. The artwork is in the style of Barcelona's Gaudi with natural lines of trails, islands of trees and a symmetry more geographic than geometric.

We soon pick up the Logone river and follow it's course. Along the banks we see the tiny beehive-shaped, rounded tents of the Arab nomads with herds of cattle and a few horses scattered along the banks. Periodically the glassy surface is broken by the smooth gliding of a dugout canoe bearing fishermen on the way to their favorite fishing holes. Some are already casting their handwoven nets in the shallow, fish-rich waters.

We follow the Logone downstream and finally see the Tandjilé snake it's way up. It joins the Logone's fast flowing waters right before Koyom and the Pentecostal Hospital. We buzz the airstrip and notice it's unusable.

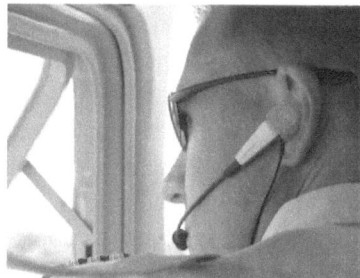

Gary

Then we pick up altitude and leave the Logone behind. The African plain becomes a distant network of fields, forests and tiny villages. A half an hour later, we pick up Tchad's other major river, the Chari. We follow it all the way to N'Djamena where the Logone and the Chari become one.

I don't even notice N'Djamena till we're right on top of it. It's just a large village lost among the trees. If it wasn't for the occasional multi-story building and the bridge across the Chari, I wouldn't have been sure it was N'Djamena. I don't think there is any other capital village in the world like Tchad's.

The airport is right across the river and has a single runway. There are two other planes pulled up at the airport. We land easily and taxi up to the MAF hangar. It is probably the world's smallest international airport. Dr. Bond flies out that evening.

It takes a few days to get visa's. Gary tries unsuccessfully to obtain permission to fly on a permanent basis in Tchad. Finally, we take off for Cameroun.

Cameroun is unremarkable for about 30 minutes until we hit the national park at Waza where we scare off some herds of antelope and giraffes. I finally feel like I'm really in Africa although some elephants and lions would be a nice touch.

As we approach Garoua we see some mountains and Gary flies us between two flat topped plateaus into a valley. The descent combined with an approaching storm and the mountains makes for a bumpy ride that threatens to loosen the tenuous hold that I've had on my breakfast since N'Djamena.

Sarah has already sent up a sickening vomit smell from the back seat. Fortunately, Gary kindly provided us with vomit bags for the flight.

I think it's hypoglycemia that's contributing to my nausea as we haven't really eaten well the last few days. At first, we couldn't find any place to stay in N'Djamena. Finally, someone opened us up a dorm room that hadn't been cleaned in months and didn't have a kitchen. So we were forced to eat off the streets, which is not easy in N'Djamena. We had to content ourselves with boiled eggs, french rolls and fish soup.

After an uneventful landing for formalities in Garoua, we take off again and head into the mountains. I'm taken in by the beauty of the rugged cliffs rising from the rich green valleys sprinkled with fields of corn and millet. I'm enchanted by the round huts with pointed thatched roofs looking like hundreds of little wizard hats on top of the rocky hills. One mountain plateau is so broad we dream aloud of building a hospital and airstrip on top of it.

Gary calls Maroua Airport to check in and the controller is shocked to hear we're going to Koza since no one has landed there in over 20 years! Gary assures her that the airstrip has been repaired.

Finally, we climb the last pass and look into Koza's valley. We approach the airstrip. I think Gary is going to land because he goes in low but we're going too fast. He's running out of airway. At the last minute he cranks the throttle and whips up over the tree tops before banking hard left and back around. Apparently, he was only looking for cows and holes that kids have dug to find mice to eat. Thanks for the warning!

We circle around again and make a very bouncy jungle strip landing without any problem. A crowd of kids runs up followed by a gang of bikers. By the time we have stopped and started to tie down two security guards from the hospital are there with sticks keeping the kids a safe two to three feet away. The crowd is so thick it is literally a sea of smiling, laughing and waving faces.

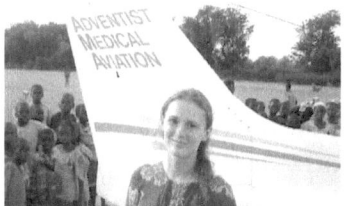

Sarah at Koza airstrip

Gary's wife Wendy drives up in Greg and Audrey Shank's pick-up truck to take us to the Koza Adventist Hospital. We are about to spend three weeks covering the medical and surgical services while Greg and Audrey cover Béré. Let the adventure begin!

10 November 2007

Esther

As I listen to Greg on the phone, I can't believe my ears. It is surreal. I don't feel panic or anything, but rather a calm, cold-blooded realization of what I need to do.

My vacation is about to be cut short.

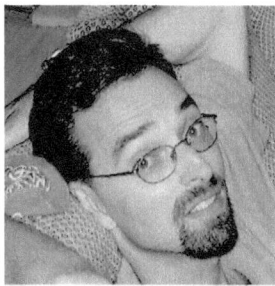

Greg

It's not really a vacation. Sarah and I have come to the Koza Adventist Hospital as part of an exchange with Drs. Greg and Audrey who are now in Béré. We have now been in Northern Cameroun for just a day over two weeks. Compared to Béré, it is a much-needed break.

In these two weeks, I've done six surgeries at Koza. Greg has done 37 at Béré. I sit around all afternoon reading and watching movies while sipping cold drinks and eating homemade ice cream. A fan and a swamp cooler are my constant companions. Meanwhile, Greg and Audrey hardly see the light of day and come home to Kerosene lamps and lukewarm tap water.

This morning, a nurse wakes me out of my electric fan-cooled sleep to see a woman in labor. I end up doing a crash C-section to save a distressed baby's life. I go home just in time for the call from Greg. His calm voice is speaking through my cell phone telling me that one of our student missionaries has severe abdominal pain and has vomited several times. Her real name is Sarah but we call her Esther because there are at least two other Sarah's around. Greg goes on to say that she has peritoneal signs and a positive Widal test for typhoid fever. She's been on IV fluids, antibiotics and morphine since yesterday. He doesn't know if she should be evacuated or what.

Fortunately, thanks to Gary Roberts and his airplane, I have the luxury of saying, "I'll be right over, let me just quickly pack my bags and I'll see you in a few hours."

It's a Saturday morning and it's going to be a long day.

I quickly go over to the church right across from the house and find Yves, the hospital administrator, to inform him of the situation. He is sitting on one of the front rows, so I drag him outside to break the news. He is understanding and wishes us a *bon voyage*. After saying good-bye to Jacques and Calda, Sarah and I pack our bags. About 30 minutes after the phone call, Gary's wife, Wendy, is driving us out to the grass airstrip.

We take down the string "fence" Gary has used to protect the plane. I detach the moorings while Gary loads up the barrels of fuel and our small backpacks. We strap ourselves in and Gary fires up the engine and the single prop roars to life. We taxi across the grass and are soon banking sharply right en route to Garoua. An uneventful landing in Garoua includes filing a flight plan and missing the immigration agents (lucky for us since we didn't have visas). Soon we are heading for Tchad. Less than three hours from Koza and we have landed in Moundou. We have a little friendly discussion (i.e. heated argument) with the customs agents ending in the usual way (laughs and hand pumping).

Twenty minutes later we are circling Béré International Airport watching Rich race down the airstrip on his motorcycle looking for goats, cows and soccer goal posts which could make our landing a little more bumpy.

"See that second path over the strip right before the little mound halfway down?" says Gary. "That's where we'll try to put down in order to miss the biggest little bump. We could circle around again, but this is faster..."

My stomach shifts somewhere over to the right as we bank sharply left and downward towards the swath cut from the Tchadian bush. Seconds later we are taxiing up to the quickly gathered crowd of kids awaiting our arrival. After the plane is unloaded, draped and secured, Rich's wife, Anne, kindly drives us over to the hospital in their Land Cruiser.

Greg is waiting for us dressed casually in jean shorts, a scrub top and large sandals. We go inside the guest house where the back room has been transformed into an intensive care of sorts. There are one patient, three doctors, three nurses, and multiple auxiliary staff (the other student missionaries) crowding around to help in any little way possible.

Sarah and I slowly enter the room. Esther gives us a weak, Morphine-duped smile and says "hi". I ask her a few questions.

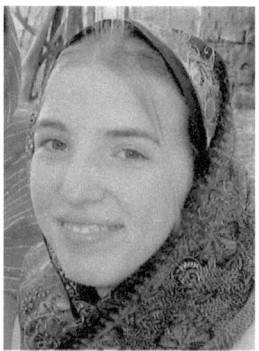

Sarah (aka Esther)

Apparently, her pain started yesterday morning early, but she thought maybe it was just part of her monthly cramps. She got on a motorcycle and took a little jaunt over to Kélo with a couple of the other volunteers. Curiously, the bumpy, bouncy ride did little to alleviate her pain. On her return, she had a typhoid test done which was sort of positive (they're sometimes hard to interpret and often have both false positives and false negatives). She was started on antibiotics and then IV fluids after she vomited. She had no urinary symptoms and bowel function was normal. She ate a little something at night. Her pain was equal on both sides of her pelvis. The pain increased with movement and tapping on the lower belly.

Greg, Audrey, Sarah and I go to the next room to discuss what to do. She has evacuation insurance and with Gary's plane we could have her in

N'Djamena maybe in time for the midnight, once-a-day flight to Paris. There is no hospital in Tchad I would prefer her to go to over ours, especially with Greg, a board-certified general surgeon on hand. We agree it could be typhoid fever, but that would usually have a longer course.

"What if it's an atypical appendicitis?" I ask. "In that case, she should be operated on as soon as possible. An evacuation won't be fast enough to keep her from perforating."

We continue to discuss. Finally, I ask Greg "If she was not a foreigner, would you operate on her?"

After a few moments, he says, "Yes, I definitely would." So that settles it. If she chooses to stay in Béré, we'll open her up.

Greg spends a long time explaining to Esther the options and she wisely calls her parents. With the time change, we at first are only able to get through to her mom who wisely tells Esther that the decision is hers. Esther doesn't take long to reply.

"Here in Béré I'm surrounded by friends and people I know. The thought of flying to Europe and being operated on far away from anyone I know...that scares me. I'd rather be operated on here...in Béré."

So, the decision is made. Hans, Sonya and Christina go to prepare the operating room and make sure everything is as clean and arranged as possible. Liz, Christina and Sarah prepare Esther for surgery.

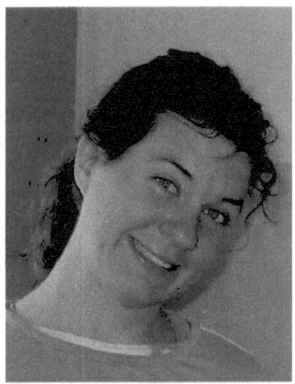

Sonya

Greg, Audrey and I wait just in the outer room of the operating theater. Once the decision is made, I am anxious to get started. Greg calms me down. We'd already waited an hour so Esther could talk to her father. At about 10:00pm we are finally ready to start.

I sit Esther up, wipe Betadine across her back, put on sterile gloves and inject a spinal anesthetic. We lay her down. Greg and I leave to respect her privacy while Audrey and the other girls prep the operating site and Audrey drapes her in sterile fashion. Greg and I scrub. When the all clear is given, we enter the operating room. Contemporary Christian praise music is going in the background as Greg and I put on our gowns and gloves. Greg moves to the left side and asks for the scalpel.

We then pray and check to see if the anesthesia has taken effect. It isn't working completely, just giving her some warm tingling feelings in her legs. Sarah gives her some Ketamine and Diazepam. When Esther is asleep, Greg slices from just below her belly button to her pubis.

As Greg enters the peritoneum, there is a small surge of liquid pus from the pelvis confirming that we've made the right decision. It just remains to be seen exactly what's the source of the infection. Greg irrigates and I suction out the pus. As I retract, Greg examines the left tube and ovary, the uterus and then the right tube and ovary. Everything is completely normal. He moves over to the cecum and as his fingers work some inflamed tissue free, out pops a very angry appendix right about to burst. With a couple quick clamps, the vessels are clamped, cut and tied. The base of the appendix is then clamped, stick tied twice and sliced off. We irrigate the abdominal cavity well and close the fascia and skin. It's taken less than an hour, the anesthesia was completely uncomplicated and we take her home to her "ICU" bed!

07 December 2007
Teenager

She is, unfortunately, one of many. Fifteen years old. A child. Tiny. Married and pregnant with a huge baby. She has been in labor for days. This morning she finally went to a health center where they tried to extract the baby with a vacuum suction applied to the baby's scalp. When that didn't work they referred her here.

It is all too common. Women usually marry as teenagers. Not just among the Muslims, but among the Nangjéré. Some even get pregnant before having their first period. Children having children. Small children having large babies that don't come out easily.

In the modern world, a woman with a small pelvis and a baby who's head is too big to come out will have a C-section. Every pregnancy thereafter, she will have excellent pre-natal care with early ultrasounds to determine the exact dates of the pregnancy. Then, an elective C-section can be performed when the fetus is mature enough and before labor begins. After three to four children, she will have a tubal ligation and live happily ever after.

In Tchad, a woman with a small pelvis and a big baby will have no prenatal visits. She'll work in the fields until labor starts. She will be transported to a mat on a dirt floor in a dark mud hut. There she will labor under the supervision of an older, experienced traditional birth attendant —sometimes for days. Then, like our girl, she may get to a health center or a hospital before dying. Often, she will be buried with her unborn child never having left the village.

Supposing, she does make it to a hospital. The well-meaning surgeon will do a C-section. Sometimes he saves the baby, but he usually just saves the mom. All is well and good. Four to five days later, the woman goes home. Often, less than a year later she is at term with her next pregnancy and labors at home. This time, her uterus has a weak spot at the area of the scar which hasn't even had time to fully heal. Maybe she'll make it to the hospital again for another C-section which will again deplete the family's meager resources. Or maybe she'll tear her uterus with the force of the contractions against the unyielding bones of her pelvis and she'll bleed to death internally.

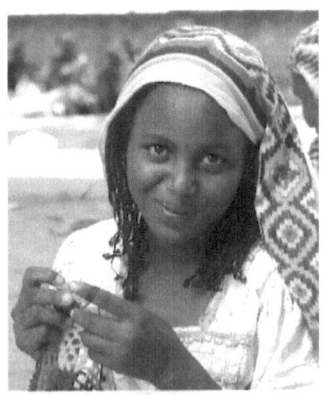

Teenage Mom

If she does make it for the second C-section, the process will repeat itself until she is either dead or abandoned by her husband as being too much of a financial drain. Who wants a woman who can only have a few kids anyway? A quarter to a half of them will probably die before the age of five, so one must have at least eight to ten kids in order to have four to six live to adulthood.

Nasara Encore

At the Béré Hospital, thanks to a technique considered brutal, archaic and cruel by the turned up noses of the western obstetrical ward, we prepare this 15 year old for a symphysiotomy.

We take her to the operating room and attach her to the monitors. She has low blood pressure and a very fast pulse. We give her antibiotics, IV fluids and call for a blood transfusion.

The problem is, she has been abandoned by her husband and most of her family. Her mom already spent most of her money at the health center. Most of what she had left she paid to put her daughter on an hour-long motorcycle ride to the hospital. Now, she only has five dollars. We can't let her die, so when the mother promises that the rest of the family are coming, we don't believe her for one instant but set her up for surgery anyway.

However, now she needs blood. Her mom is not a match. We don't have a blood bank and rely on family members to donate. None of our volunteer staff is compatible either. We are forced to do our best without blood.

I shave and prep the pubic area. I inject 10ml of local anesthetic. Abel has placed a urinary catheter. IV fluids are running. Heart rate is 140 and blood pressure 80/40. I slice down to the cartilage and with my other hand displacing the urinary catheter inside, I slowly incise the fibers from top to bottom being careful not to enter the bladder or vagina. Abel and Siméon have the legs flexed and externally rotated. On cue from me, they spread the legs down and the pelvis pops open with a load "crack".

As blood gushes out of the wound, I stuff two gauze pads down to stem the bleeding. I cut an episiotomy and apply our own vacuum delivery device to the head. She has no strength left to push and the baby's scalp won't hold the vacuum. The head still won't come out.

I ask Siméon to put some Oxytocin in the IV fluids and to open it wide up. Slowly, the uterus contracts and pushes the head out little by little as I gently tug with the vacuum on the baby's head. Finally, the head pops out with a gush of thick dark meconium. The neck is strangulated with a tight nuchal cord that I can barely slide over the head. Finally, the shoulders and arms slip out and the rest of the body slides out quickly.

I check the umbilical pulse. Nothing. The baby has been dead for a while. The placenta quickly follows thanks to the Oxytocin still running and her uterus forms up nicely. She's bleeding quite a bit from where I cut the episiotomy. I stuff in a bunch of gauze sponges and then pull out the sponges from the symphysiotomy wound.

I irrigate the wound and close it in two layers. I then suture up the episiotomy. She continues to bleed. Siméon checks her hemoglobin: 5.1 g/dl. Very low. Still no blood for transfusion.

I check all inside and finally find a tear up around her urethra. When I suture it the bleeding finally stops. She is sweating and a little delirious. Heart rate still 140s and blood pressure 90/50 now after several liters of fluid. We have no choice but to send her out to the ward and hope the family members come quickly.

That evening, at about 8:00pm, Liz comes to talk to me about several patients. She mentions that the symphysiotomy girl has low blood pressure, a fast heart rate and now a fever of 40° C. She is wavering in and out of consciousness and is sweating profusely.

I tell Liz to give her injectable Chloramphenical, a Quinine drip and a fluid bolus. After Liz leaves, I take a long drink of water and something impels me to go see her myself.

I find her like Liz said. She is almost in fatal shock. Only blood will help. I help Liz get the medicines and IV fluids going.

The mother keeps wringing her hands and asking *"Loe ne mega? Loe ne mega?"* What's going on? What's going on? I tell her *"Koubra kang ddi"* There is no blood. She runs off. Liz and I continue our work.

The mother soon comes back with the brother of another patient, a young man who just had his leg amputated. He's been with us for several weeks. The brother and another man say they are willing to donate blood. The other man just gave a pint for his relative two days ago but is willing to give again. We find his blood isn't a match.

Then we think of Allison, the volunteer at the Evangelical Mission who's staying with us for a week while Rich and Anne are in N'Djamena. We call her and both she and the brother of the amputee are compatible. People don't just give blood to non-relatives, but this man is encouragingly different, going against the cultural pressure and ignorance we are surrounded with to save the life of a stranger.

After two units of blood, the next morning the girl is a different person. She is up moving around with normal vital signs and has eaten some porridge for breakfast. Her uterus is firm, the wounds look good and she is hardly spotting at all.

Liz comes in at 5:00am the following morning to start her Quinine drip and finds her cold and stiff. Four family members are around her and haven't noticed. Liz informs them and they begin the death wail immediately, bundle up the corpse and head home.

2008

16 January 2008

Stone

I slip on my white coat over my scrubs and Snapper Jack's sweatshirt—believe it or not, it does get cold in Tchad—lock up my office and head out to the wards.

I walk through the wards and notice a crowd lounging around outside. I exit quickly shouting in French, "Rounds are starting! Everyone who's with a patient come in, all other visitors leave!"

I accompany my shouts with a few aggressive gestures and repeat myself a lot while the nurses translate my rustic French into Arabic and Nangjéré. After about 15 minutes, almost everyone not supposed to be inside the hospital compound has cleared out. The hospital enjoys a rare moment of relative tranquility.

Not for long.

The wards are even more crowded than usual. The pediatric ward and emergency room have been vacated so the leaky roof and moth-eaten ceiling can be replaced. As a result, even more patients are crammed into the already over-burdened wards.

I start with Pediatrics. Tchibtchang gathers the charts and calls the nursing students. The charge nurse, Jacob, joins us along with Camilla, the Danish medical student and we start rounding on the kids.

I come to the last of the pediatric patients, a skinny ten year old boy with bulging eyes staring at us blankly. Suddenly, he repeats his performance of yesterday. I was so non-plussed then, that I called the chaplain to see if he could figure out if the child was demon-possessed.

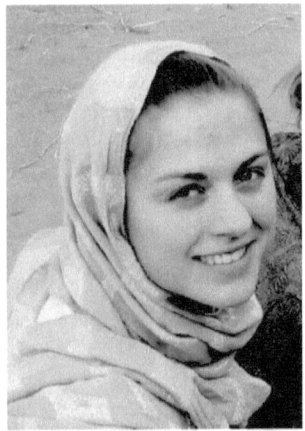

Camilla

The boy somehow manages to combine three extraordinary moves into one well-polished fluid motion apparently perfected by years of repetition. He accompanies the maneuver with a blood-curdling scream like a banshee being bit by a thousand bees.

In one simultaneous gesture the boy flips from his back to a kneeling position, thrusts his butt up into the air, reaches his hand around his back, sticks his index finger into his anus, and releases a stream of urine that would make a race-horse proud while his penis thrashes around like a fire hose out of control. All the time he writhes around like a cat in a bag and yells like someone is slowly skinning him alive.

I'm shocked and unnerved. I quickly grab his arms removing his hand from his butt, flip him over and pin him to the urine soaked mattress. I notice the urine is tinged with pus. I ask for his lab results as he moans, groans and struggles uselessly. His stool test is normal and his urine not surprisingly shows an abundance of white blood cells.

I decide to do a rectal exam. I quickly call for a glove and feel inside the child's rectum. Where his prostate should be is a large, hard, smooth mass that is somewhat oblong moving towards his bladder.

An ultrasound confirms a calcified mass in his bladder.

An hour later I poise over the boy's lower abdomen with a scalpel as Abel prays. A few slices later and I'm in his bladder. Even though I kind of expect it, chills still run up and down my spine. My arm hairs stand on end as I reach a gloved finger into the bladder and touch the large urinary calculus.

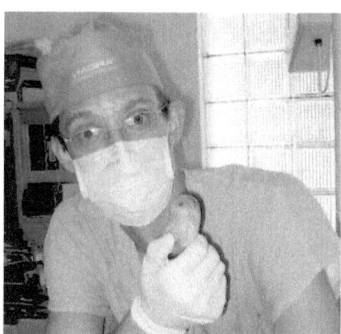

James & bladder stone

It's so large compared to the small kid's bladder that it is quite difficult to extract. I finally open the wound more and slip some forceps around it and squeeze it out like a difficult childbirth. There on the table before me is an three inch by one inch long kidney bean-shaped stone.

After closing the bladder and skin, I realize that the boy is actually quite smart and creative after all. The weight of the stone caused urinary obstruction through gravity pulling it down to block the urinary outlet. When his bladder got so full he couldn't stand the pressure of the retention, he flipped over with his buttocks in the air so gravity and a well-placed rectal finger would push the stone off the exit releasing a high pressure urinary stream bringing relief but causing excruciating pain at the same time.

Who know's how long he's suffered with this? The parents say he's been like this all his life despite going to many hospitals and spending months as an inpatient. I'm just thankful God insisted I do a rectal exam.

22 January 2008
Stumbling

I stumble through the dark as I pull on my socks, lace up my shoes and slip on my sweatshirt. As I open the gate I almost trip over a pile of human excrement. The darkness is almost complete. Only an occasional star sneaks through the thick layer of angry clouds.

A dry, icy desert wind is blowing across the plain chilling me to the bone.

As my eyes adjust I can barely make out the faintest trace of the path where the white sand makes a slight distinction between itself and the dark flora of the Sahel.

I start to jog hesitantly as I fight to keep from tripping and falling. The only thing breaking the monotony of the obscurity are two dark red glows of distant brush fires illuminating the horizon like a dragon's nostrils.

I wonder if I can find the way.

My thoughts begin to tumble on themselves like stones forever caught in the undertow of a river's eddy:

A seven day old born at home, probably on a dirt floor with a razor blade and some old twine to take care of the umbilical cord. Now I see him in my mind: face pinched, eyes squinting, hand clenched, lost forever in the dark clutches of tetanus.

A woman, almost unconscious, breathing fast and shallow, her pregnant belly tender and swollen with blood and a dead fetus from a ruptured uterus. A C-section and hysterectomy later she is rapidly being transfused to desperately save her life. A week later I have her belly open again in front of me with intestines glued together with the destructive inflammation of blood clots. Multiple blood transfusions later I'm forced to open her skin wound to let out the post operative infection.

A small girl with a swollen belly returns to see us after two successful courses of treatment for Burkitt's lymphoma, but who decided to not come back for her further doses and now has a spleen and pelvis filled with knotty tumors.

A tall, striking 19 year old HIV-positive woman comes back with her one and a half year old AIDS baby who's bloody diarrhea just won't let up. Her husband is out of town on "business".

A slender, beautiful eleven year old is back hospitalized after the surgery to remove her rotting lower leg bone sticking out wasn't complete enough to remove the year old infection.

A 22 year old woman with a small baby dies of heart failure due to a heart rhythm disturbance we are unable to diagnose and treat due to lack of equipment and medication.

Another seven-day-old has parents who refuse to let her be hospitalized with fever and a swollen belly and then bring her back one day later on death's door hoping we can work a miracle.

Five hernia patients wait patiently outside the operating theater.

A woman is referred from a health center two days after being diagnosed with appendicitis and treated with aspirin and worm medicine.

A man comes in with small, non-itchy blisters all over his body and is found to have HIV and syphilis.

Drums, drums in the deep pound out a solemn, enchanting rhythm through the night as wails and shrieks waft over the village of Béré like sulfurous trails of smoke below piercing red eyes.

And all I've been thinking about only happened yesterday as I stumble once again through the pre-dawn darkness.

I stop by a twisted, gnarled, stunted tree trunk with a few branches and scattered leaves. I pause to stretch and as I do the sadness, frustration, fear and inadequacy that has been exploding out in shocking anger now bursts on the scene in deep, uncontrollable sobs as the tears pour down my cheeks.

I continue on, straining to see the road ahead, trying to cry as my out of shape lungs suck in the dry, cool air. My hands are deep in my sleeves and my hood is up desperately trying to chase out the chill.

I pass the first great tree and then turn around at the second according to my ritual. The path back is a little clearer. A steel grey sky is starting to peer through the clouds. I pick up speed as I head for home.

The dawn is about to break.

31 January 2008
Couscous & Goat

The couscous steamed in the belly of the goat is quite tasty if a little undercooked. I spoon another mouthful of the dish garnished with a piece of flesh ripped off the greasy leg bone on my plate. How else would one welcome someone as important as the Minister of Health?

The morning starts off with trying to desperately tear myself out of bed. I'm exhausted. I've done 80 plus surgeries this month including 24 in a five day stretch last week. As the same time, I'm working on cleaning out the inside of the ambulance that looks like it had been used as storage for any spare part containing massive amounts of old oil.

Sarah has warmed up the Danish cauliflower gravy over yesterday's mashed potatoes and fake meat dish. Our nurse, Job, exhorts us in morning worship from Acts 13 and we talk about quinine drips for kids in staff meeting.

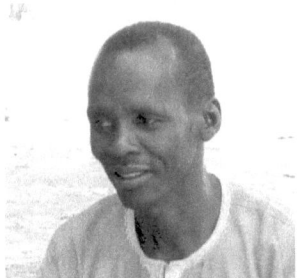

Job

It's during this encounter that someone calls to say that the Minister of Health will be driving through Béré at 11:00am and could we please all be there to welcome him?

Sure, no problem, is that 11 o'clock African time?

I spend some time with André and Noel discussing the spiritual battle facing us and how we can help each other to keep from being taken out by our enemy.

As I head to the operating room for the first case, Sarah corners me as I pass the door to the temporary ER.

"Could you come see this patient? He has peritonitis."

Unfortunately, she's right. He's had pain for a week, severe since this morning accompanied by vomiting. He jumps and grimaces when I tap on his belly. There is tenderness inside when I do a rectal exam.

His wife pays for the surgery and we wheel him in. The 20-year-old woman born without a vagina, the old man with the hernia and the even older man who can't pee because of his huge prostate will have to wait for their elective surgeries.

Within 20 minutes of diagnosis, my knife is slicing through skin, muscle, fat, blood vessels, fascia and peritoneum to let out a bubbly gush of slimy green fluid over some angry, blotched loops of small intestine.

I enlarge the incision to the sternum with scissors and after sucking up all the goo I find the small hole in his stomach letting it all out. It's a perforated peptic ulcer.

I put in some silk sutures along the perforation but don't tie them. Then I drag in a piece of omentum and tie it over the hole with the sutures. I then irrigate, wash, rinse, aspirate and close up.

It's only 11:00am. Since it's African time, maybe I have time for a prostate before going to meet the Minister.

Abel and Siméon make a super efficient operating room team. They soon have the patient out, the operating room cleaned and the grandpa sitting on the table ready for his spinal anesthetic almost before I turn around.

As soon as the lidocaine is in his spinal canal we lay him down, lower the head of the table, strap him in, and prep his abdomen and groin with Betadine. Camilla, the Danish medical student, scrubs with me.

After Abel's prayer, I cut down horizontally to the bladder and incise it vertically letting out a stream of blood tinged urine. Camilla grabs the suction catheter and keeps the field clean while I enlarge the bladder incision. Siméon pulls out the foley catheter while I stick my finger in to feel the mass of prostate bulging into the bladder.

I insert my index finger into the prostate where the urine should normally go out and with the pressure of the finger tip start to shell out the prostate. I sweep around. My fingers start to cramp from the pressure and awkward position as my body twists and contorts over the patient trying to get my finger in deep enough to go all the way around the enormous adenoma.

Finally, the prostate pops out and I fish it out of the bladder. Siméon inserts the large three-way foley catheter that I guide through the crater left where the prostate should be. Camilla suctions up the blood that wells up while Siméon inserts 30mL into the ballon to tamponade off the bleeding.

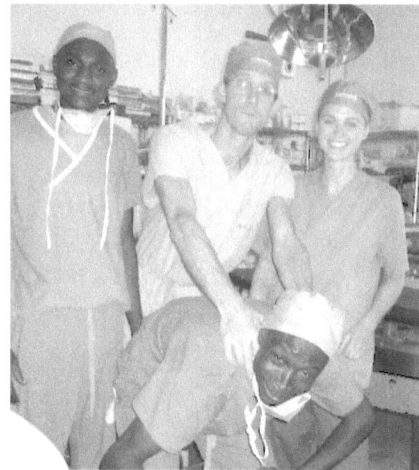

Siméon, James, Abel & Camilla

I suture the bladder, fascia and skin. Siméon starts the bladder irrigation running as blood-tinged fluid flows out into the urine bag. It's only 12:34pm and I might have time to catch the Minister of Health.

Sonya and I walk over to the District Medical Office where a convoy of seven cars is parked along the main street in the red dirt of Béré. A group of raggedy Red Cross volunteers, each with a unique red cross painted on his shirt, collects outside the offices. Out back under the mango tree the VIPs gather.

I pass the camouflage-wearing, turban-toting soldier with his AK47, go through the chainlink and sit on the edge of a chair next to my wife. In the low slung, neon green, fake velvet chair of honor is a simply dressed, tall, sunglasses-wearing Tchadian I assume is the Minister of Health.

A camera man makes sure to video the proceedings as two woman come in bearing the two couscous stuffed goats on platters, anatomy complete minus the heads. A greasy finger-stuffing, soda-popping 15 minutes later the Minister gets up for his speech.

"We have been touring the country to get a better idea of the conditions that you, our frontline health care workers, work under. We've been all over the south-central region for a week seeing hospitals from Doba to Koumra to Sarh to Lai and now Béré.

"There are less than 400 physicians in all of Tchad, less than 4000 nurses and less than 200 midwives. This is why Tchad has some of the worst maternal child statistics in the world."

With that and some other encouraging words, they take their leave. They are in a hurry since word has come this morning that the united rebel forces are already in Ati vowing to take N'djamena and overthrow the President.

No one is worried too much yet because European Union special forces have started arriving since yesterday and the rebels aren't strong enough. At least no one is fleeing N'Djamena yet for the bush which everyone takes as a good sign.

So I return to round on the hospitalized patients. Later, I schedule another hernia and a vaginal hysterectomy for prolapsed uterus that is completely outside the woman's body. The nurses call me to see a baby who needs a spinal tap. I draw out cloudy spinal fluid on an infant already struggling with malaria and severe anemia, prescribe antibiotics and head home.

Even after the couscous and goat I still crave some of my wife's Danish home-cooking.

06 February 2008
Slick

I'm sitting peacefully at home when Tchibtchang comes to see me.

"A young pregnant woman just arrived in a coma. Her blood pressure is high, she has a fever and we can't find the baby's heartbeat."

I give some instructions for further tests, put her on a quinine drip and hope it isn't pre-eclampsia.

The next morning, I see her during rounds. She is writhing around in bed with four people trying to hold her down. The nurses show me the results of the urine protein and it's negative for pre-eclampsia. She has a slightly positive malaria smear. I continue her quinine drip. I check the fetal heartbeat myself and confirm that the baby is indeed already dead. I then order some medicine to stimulate labor and hopefully deliver the stillborn child.

All day long she moans, thrashes and screams.

That evening Salomon comes to see me about the same patient. The woman is in the delivery room lying half naked on the table with her mom and aunt holding her arms and legs to keep her from pulling out her IV.

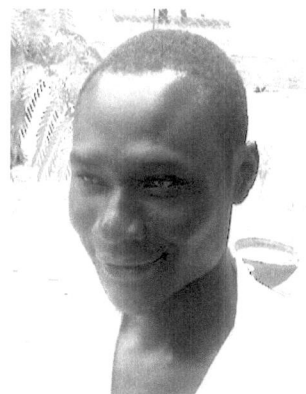
Salomon

"She is crying as if being tortured," says Salomon in French. "It's all we can do to keep her from biting herself and falling to the floor."

I go in and confirm what Salomon told me. I check her abdomen and she isn't having good enough contractions so I turn up the Oxytocin drip. The thoughts that start to come into my mind I try to ignore, but finally I blurt out:

"I think she's being harassed by evil spirits!"

Salomon translates into Ngambai for the family. Through Salomon's interpretation we discuss what that means and how the only treatment is prayer because no amount of drips, medications or even surgery can exorcise a demon.

Salomon prays long and hard in Ngambai. I finish with a prayer in French begging God to keep his promise that he came to deliver the prisoners and set the captives free. A few minutes later she is calm and snoring. I leave and go home.

Salomon soon comes to get me to see her again. I enter the delivery room and find an even wilder patient. As the woman thrashes around on the table we try to keep her from falling to the ground and from biting herself. She has delivered the still-born and now the placenta has been stuck for 45 minutes. She is stiffening her legs, lolling her head and wildly waving her arms as we try to hold on. However, with all the blood smeared everywhere she is as slick as a greased watermelon in a swimming pool.

I put on some gloves and try to reach inside to pull out the placenta but she clamps her legs together. The women are shouting at her in Ngambai and I'm trying to pry her leg apart with one arm as I try to grab the placenta with the other. Finally, frustrated, I reach up and grab her chin and shake her.

"Let me help you!" I scream.

She calms a little letting me get my hand in the uterus, grab the placenta and pull it out before all hell breaks loose again. Now she starts to bleed heavily.

"Get me some Oxytocin and Methergine quick!" I yell.

Liz and Sonya rush to get them. I try to hold on to the patient as the blood coursing from within makes her more and more slippery. The thrashing has spattered her legs, back and belly with blood. I try to massage her ritually scarred abdomen but her powerful rectus muscles are contracted as she resists with all her might.

Without time to think and scared that this demon is trying to kill her by keeping me from stopping the bleeding I reach up and slap her face. I shake her again while pleading with her to let me help. She calms a little and starts asking "Khalas? Khalas?" (Is it finished? Is is over?)

I'm able to massage her uterus and it starts to firm up a little. Then she starts to thrash around again and I'm forced to press my fist down between her rectal muscles to keep pressure on the uterus.

Sonya comes back with the Methergine and Oxytocin but the intramuscular shots start an even crazier bout of thrashing. Finally, we give her some Chlorpromazine to try and calm her. At last, the bleeding slows down. It's 3:30am and I've been with her for 45 minutes. I come back to the house, plug in some quiet music.

I'm drained but not discouraged.

The next day, Salomon tells me that they've finally discovered why she was possessed. Apparently, even though she never went to the witch doctor herself, her relatives went to a sorcerer to find out why she was sick and were told that someone had put a fetish curse on her. I refer her to our chaplain, Noel, for further spiritual care.

22 February 2008
Update

Fortunately, the fighting in Tchad never came close to Béré but stayed in N'Djamena. Now things have calmed down and are back to "normal" even in the capital.

Sarah and I are in Denmark starting our furlough. We left a few weeks earlier than planned, not due to the rebel activity in Tchad but due to personal burn-out. We hope and pray this furlough will renew our strength allowing us to return to Tchad.

We are encouraged by a surgeon, Dr. Bond, who has committed to working a year in Béré. If we could just find one more physician of any specialty to help us then the prospects are indeed bright for the future of the Béré Adventist Hospital. Sarah and I hope to continue our dream of dedicating our lives to working in Tchad.

12 April 2008
Infertility

Sarah and I drive through the narrow streets of Aalborg. We've been in Denmark for six weeks. Two different ski trips to Norway have helped us to start recovering from our burnout. The first trip was with the Cafekirken in Copenhagen and the second with our friends Karsten and Giske from Vejlefjord.

Now we are looking for the doctor's office. Neither one of us is sick, we just haven't been able to have kids. The doctor is a fertility specialist. We take the stairs up to the second floor of a downtown high rise and enter a modern looking doctor's office.

Sarah approaches the secretary and speaks to her in Danish. I go into the glassed-in waiting room and leaf through some magazines. Sarah joins me. A few minutes later, the secretary pokes her head in and speaks in English.

"Anders is ready to see you now."

I'm struck by the informality. No Doctor so-and-so or other titles. Everyone is on first name basis. It's part of the Danish concept of *janteloven* meaning the worst thing one can do in Danish culture is think one is better than someone else.

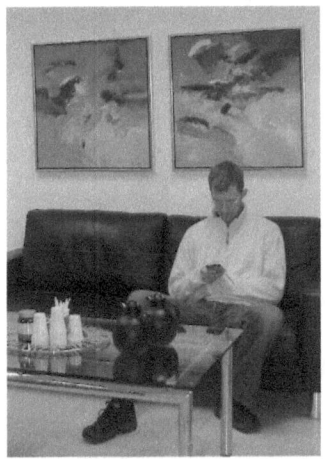

James at the fertility clinic

As if to prove the point, Anders comes out to meet us dressed in jeans and a polo shirt. He has no white coat, stethoscope, name badge or anything at all that might identify him as a physician.

The interview is laid-back and Anders sends us off to do some tests. After a week, we are back to see him to get the results.

"We haven't found anything wrong. You have what's called unexplained infertility. The treatment is in vitro fertilization or IVF."

Sarah gets a prescription for some medicine and we start the process. We'll have to wait and see if it works.

20 May 2008
Farcha

As I step out of the plane the heat hits me smack in the face. The hazy orange, low lit airstrip of the Hassan Djamous International airport rises to meet me as I descend the portable stairs onto the tarmac. A brief passport and visa check later and I'm waiting for my bags which never arrive.

Odei, Hans and our new driver, Levi, are there to meet us. My sister Chelsey and the team from Florida is with Sarah and I. Everyone else's bags has arrived so we load up the truck. Rick, Hans and I climb in the back on top of the luggage for a dimly lit ride through downtown N'Djamena to the mission guest house at TEAM.

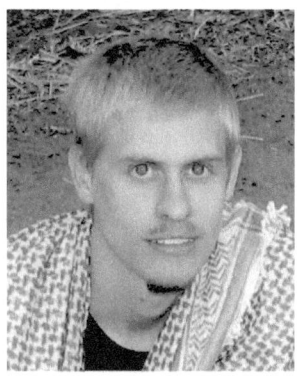
Hans

After some spaghetti and watermelon, I take a cold shower to try and cool down a little. By not drying off and letting the fan evaporate the water on my skin I am able to at least lie down and sleep fitfully. By 6:00am I can no longer sleep and the sheets are soaked with my sweat.

True to his promise, Odei is there to meet me at 8:30am to take me to his church in Farcha. A homemade drum set fashioned out of various tin cans and scraps of metal welded together and covered with goat skins guides the three different choirs in their diverse African chants. The rhythms course through my blood bringing me into an awareness of the divine.

Afterwards, Odei and I hop on his motorcycle and swerve through the dips and humps of the unpaved city streets towards the district hospital. One of his friends has been hospitalized that week. We first pull over to a shack made of woven reeds where a 12-year-old boy is selling water in a bag. We rip open the edges and guzzle half a liter each down our parched throats.

To turn into the hospital we must carefully navigate a ditch filled with putrid water and covered in slime. A variety of bottles and cans struggle desperately to stay above the surface as the gunk relentlessly tugs them under. We turn past a rickety, iron framed chain link gate hanging off a couple of badly attached hinges and into the small courtyard of the District Hospital of Farcha.

Peeling yellow paint, twisted hand rails and crumbly cement steps lead us past a few customers lounging on torn mats under the shade of a few gnarled bushes almost resembling trees. The well-tiled hallway branches immediately off left and right while straight ahead is a tiny courtyard filled with plastic bags, IV tubing and littered with paper that has all tumbled off a pile of trash from an overstuffed metal barrel that has been cut in half.

Some Tchadians wearing white coats means that there are a few nurses present. Odei greets several of them and we are oriented down the dimly lit hall to the left. We peer into a dark room filled with a few beds, some with mattresses. Lots of visitors wearing brightly colored robes and head scarves stare up at us. There are a few patients hooked up to IVs suspended from windows, a couple of rickety IV poles and even off the ceiling.

Someone informs us that Odei's friend is outside. We head to the back where some stray dogs scrounge through the piles of refuse around the smoky outdoor kitchen. We finally find our man under a tree with a few buddies. After some extended greetings and joking around we discover that he has malaria which is being being partially treated. But he also has a chronic cough for weeks and no one has tested him for tuberculosis. We give some suggestions, chat some more and finally get up to leave.

The next day, we leave early from N'Djamena and arrive in Béré in the afternoon. Our poor hospital doesn't seem so bad after the shock of the Farcha Hospital.

26 May 2008

HIV premie

I tried to tell her. I warned her so many times. But she just wanted to do what felt right in the moment. She just wanted to have a baby.

She's only a child still herself: 19-years-old but looks 13 or 14. She has AIDS and has already been treated for eight months for tuberculosis and is on antiretroviral therapy. She's unmarried.

Now, she sits in my office cradling affectionately a tiny premature baby boy. All the books on HIV management tell me that if possible, the baby should not be breast fed, but formula fed to avoid the risk of HIV infection through the milk. However, this tiny, malnourished life needs all the help it can get.

Despite her obvious thrill at being a mom and holding a baby in her arms, she has no clue what taking care of this baby will mean or how to help it grows up healthy and HIV-free. She has been underfeeding him, feeding him only "when he's hungry."

"So he tells you when he's hungry?" I gently chide trying to use humor to get her to realize it's her responsibility to feed him regularly whether he wants it or not.

It does seem she is doing some things right. She washes and boils the bottle and uses only clean water to mix the formula. I tell her to continue the formula, but decide to hospitalize her so she can get help with the idea of regular feedings and what's the appropriate amount.

Of course, nurses who are trained to suture, treat emergencies, deliver babies, give shots and start IVs—like our locals—haven't been exposed to the other side of nursing: patient education, daily needs assessment, nutrition, etc.

As I look into the gaunt, yet strangely peaceful and trusting face of this four pound premie, I fear his days are numbered.

28 May 2008

Fracture

The man is lying on the twisted gurney in obvious pain. His relatives and friends stand around panting, trying to catch their breath. They've just hauled him in off the back of the pick-up where he had bounced up, down and all around on the pothole-filled dirt road from Lai.

I bend over his left leg and gently lift the blood soaked rags. A Betadine browned compress with a bright red bloody center is all that stands between me and the fracture. I gingerly lift it up to see the bright white shard of bone sticking up from a black spider-webbed mass of sutures ineffectively attempting to hold the wound together.

It's been three days since he fell off the gravel truck.

A piece of cardboard is bent around the back and sides of the legs and tied on with string in a lame effort to stabilize the broken tibia.

"We have to operate, clean out the wound and try to get the fracture stabilized," I inform the family.

The family understands and willing forks over the 30,000 francs necessary for the surgery, anesthesia, medications and hospital stay.

After knocking him out with a heavy dose of Ketamine and Valium I have my sister Chelsey grab his foot and pull.

"Lean into it, let your body weight do the work, not your arms," I coach her.

Siméon is at the head of the gurney. We are in the operating room prep room with a pulse oximeter attached to monitor our anesthetized patient. Siméon has just given the antibiotics.

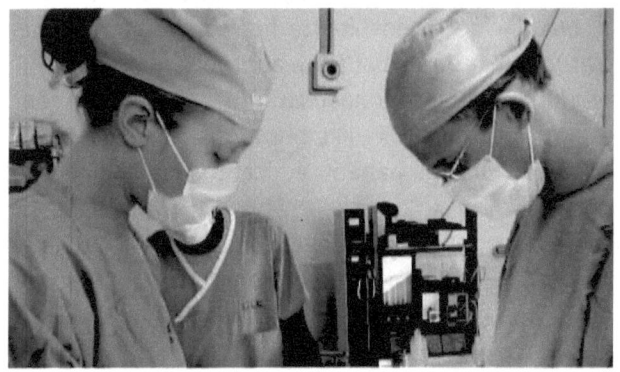

Chelsey & James

I prepare a five liter basin of diluted bleach solution and open up a tray of sterile instruments. The procedure is not sterile as the sand and gravel inside the wound testify, but I guess sterile-to-start-with instruments isn't a bad idea.

I cut all the old sutures and bend the foot down and back so the bone fragment sticks out more allowing me to put my finger behind the bone and with the help of a bulb syringe start to wash out the debris.

After five liters of irrigation, the wound is fairly clean. I cut off the dead looking tissue and then try and reduce the fracture. A huge posterior piece of the bone is not there, probably removed in Lai, meaning the bone is trying to balance itself on the half centimeter anterior segment. It doesn't work very well but with Siméon now pulling and Chelsey putting medial pressure on the lower segment and lateral pressure on the upper segment it stays pretty well.

Then I have to try and close a gaping 10 cm wound. I use heavy suture with special mattress type sutures and little by little it mostly closes but under a lot of tension. Who knows if it'll hold up, but it's the best I can do. Then, I pull out an external hard plastic shell for lower leg fractures and strap it around the leg to stabilize the fracture.

Amazingly, three days later, the wound is still holding together with no signs of infection and the fracture is more or less still in a good orientation to heal. Maybe a miracle will happen.

15 June 2008
Flashlights

I'm bouncing along the supposedly paved streets of N'Djamena. The Hilux pickup that André wrecked has somehow been revived. It's so thrashed-looking, though, that you wouldn't believe it could still be running unless you've lived in Tchad. I never cease to be amazed by the miracles Tchadian mechanics can perform to keep the majority of Tchadian vehicles limping along the highways and byways of the African plain.

Sitting next to me is Enock, a squat, heavily muscled man slowly turning into a fat nursing student. He flashes a toothy grin complete with a glint off a gold tipped tooth. As we chat, he tells me the following unbelievable story.

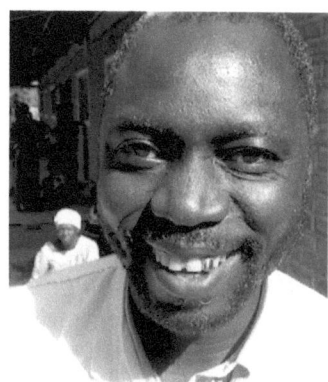

Enock

Several years ago, his son became deathly ill with severe abdominal pain. He was rushed to the health center who appropriately referred him to the National Reference Hospital in N'Djamena. They were fortunately living there at the time and were able to get him in quickly.

It was the middle of the night. Trying to maneuver through the crazy ER with people piled all over the place already cost him some "tea" and "soap" money but finally he was seen by a doctor who confirmed the diagnosis: acute appendicitis. He was scheduled for surgery that very night.

As Enock and his wife huddled together praying, the surgery team wheeled their son away through the swinging doors on a gurney. All they could do was sit and wait. Half hour later, all the lights went out.

Of course, there was instant confusion and they heard an orderly fumbling through the halls and bursting through the doors of the operating room. In a frantic rush he bumped into Enock.

"Are you the father of the boy with appendicitis?" He demanded.

"Yes, what's going on?"

"We're in the middle of the case, your son's belly is open and we have no light."

"Yeah, I noticed...what...?"

"Hurry out to the market and buy some flashlights...HURRY!"

Enock rushed out, down the stairs, out the door of the hospital, hailed a motorcycle taxi, raced to the market, luckily found someone open, bought two flashlights and hurried back.

The surgeons then continued their life saving procedure and a week later Enock's son was home safe and sound.

Only in Tchad.

17 June 2008

Window

Thunder rolls. A cool breeze bursts through the window ruffling the papers on the table. I'm sitting, staring out my window at life in Béré as the sun goes down behind the house. The red sunset reflects off the mango tree leaves poking up like heads of broccoli above the pale tan of the mud brick walls of my neighbors lots. The thatch roofs of the huts add no color but rather texture and ruggedness. A gentle rain sprinkles down. The sky is a steel grey.

People pass by on the path that runs 20 feet from where I sit behind mosquito screen and iron bars. Finally, a little rest from a long 24 hours of hospital work.

It started yesterday evening after the generator came on bringing us a few hours of light. A man presents with a simple testicular abscess that we drain in the operating room by removing his testicle.

Tchibtchang then calls me to see an old man with urinary retention. He had gone to a health center where they tried to insert a catheter into his bladder but couldn't get it in. They referred him to us. I see him now with a huge round mass in his lower abdomen: a distended bladder holding a liter or two of urine. I try half-heartedly for a few minutes knowing that a false track has probably been created leaving me with no option except to drain his bladder through his abdominal wall.

Then, I remember an instrument I saw among the bag of weird, mostly useless instruments brought by one of our volunteers. I hurry home and come back with an instrument looking like a torture device from the dark ages. It's a metal tube with a tee at the end. Perpendicular to the tee a spout curves out. On top is a round ball on a piston connected to a four-sided razor sharp spearhead poking out the opposite end.

I inject some local anesthetic above the pubic bone of the old gentleman, make a small skin incision and then poke and twist the torture device straight in until I feel a "pop". I pull back the piston and bloody, foul-smelling urine jets out the spout all over the bed and partly in the basin we'd arranged for it to go in. I then slide a rubber tube down the spout into the bladder and pull the torture device out. I tie the tube in place and attach it to a drain bag. I send him to the ward after examining his prostate with a gloved finger and confirming that it's monstrously enlarged.

Outside my window, a fat lady waddles on by shoving a push cart. Chickens peck the ground looking for insects while trying to escape the amorous advances of a strutting, cocky rooster.

Last night at 11:00pm, another old man comes in with urinary retention. He tells the same story as the first man: he went to a health center, they tried to put in catheter, got blood instead of urine, and sent him to the hospital. This time I'm ready and quickly repeat the same supra-pubic insertion of the drainage tube under local anesthetic with the severe-looking trocar.

The rain continues to fall outside as a woman walks her friend out the gate of her courtyard half way down her path to the main path. As the saying goes here in Tchad, if I accompany you out then my blessing goes with you. She stops and shakes hands and her tall lanky friend saunters away down the path glancing casually around and greeting the two boys bringing the cows back in from grazing. A sharp smack with a long stick ensures that the cows keep up a healthy trot and stay in line.

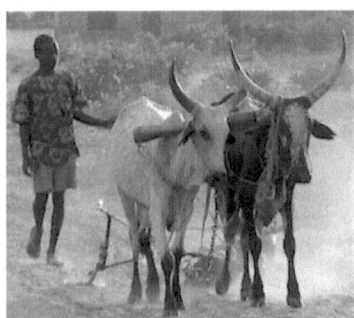

Tchadian cattle

The morning brings a pair of hernias. Not too unusual except that both have associated hydroceles. We do them with the generator running, but since it's kind of a mutant, handicapped generator, it can only do a few things at a time so we operate using ambient light so we can run the air conditioner. As it is, sweat flows freely down the sleeves of my gown and into my gloves.

In between cases, a ten year old boy comes in after being attacked by a bull on the outside of his upper arm. A superficial 10cm U-shaped wound looks like it was cut with a knife or razor blade. How he avoided massive injury with those big horns I'll never know. I suture him up under general anesthesia and then do the second hernia and hydrocele combo.

A few hours later, another ten year old boy comes in with a wound to his armpit from another bull's horn. This one is also superficial having missed his blood vessels and lungs. Those bulls need to practice their goring if they want to be taken seriously. I let Siméon suture this one up while I grab a bite to eat.

A large woman saunters by outside my house as I sit and take in the calm evening scene around my house. On her head are carefully balance an enormous pile of bound reeds. I'll never cease to be amazed. Where this path joins the main road in front of the hospital a group of about six kids hop, skip and talk animatedly to each other as they head away from me. A tiny girl in a tattered pink dress does semi-cartwheels, her bare feet flailing in the air before tumbling over on her back.

As I'm about to go home a little after 3:00pm, one of the nurses comes to tell me that one of the kids on pediatrics is pooping blood. I go over to see one of the kids we'd treated for meningitis and malaria. She'd also got a blood transfusion for anemia. She was doing better this morning according to the family and had finished the treatment. She always looked a little drowsy to me, but I guess I just chocked it up to being worn out from all that's happened.

She is four-months-old, very cute, and with devoted parents.

She is resting face down on her mom's lap, butt cheeks in the air, legs hanging down and dark red, partially coagulated blood coming out of her anus. In medical school they told us about something called "red currant jelly stool." Now, I've finally seen what they're talking about. I am suspicious of intussusception and confirm my suspicions with a quick look in my books. Her small intestine has been swallowed by her large intestine and now is getting necrotic.

We take her to the operating room. She looks so tiny on that large table. She only weighs a little over 10 lbs. Abel finds an IV, Siméon administers the anesthetic and after prayer I open up the thin skin of her belly with much trepidation.

Some red inflammatory fluid bubbles out along with most of her small intestines. I search for where her small intestine joins her large bowel and don't find what I expect. Instead, I find a deep red, almost black gangrenous appendix that fortunately hasn't ruptured. I perform an appendectomy and close up her abdomen.

As I hand her back to her parents, tubes coming out from all over, I can't help but hope that one day soon, she too will be attempting cartwheels down the streets of Béré.

22 June 2008
Moundou

Sarah and I are in Tchad's second largest city, Moundou. We've come here with Pastor Job, my old friend from the Adventist Mission. We'd been noticing in Béré that a lot of patients are coming from urban

Moundou to very rural Béré to have surgery. I want to know why. I've already visited the one hospital in town and it's in sad shape.

Now, Job wants to show me an old mission house that's fallen into the hands of the military. It was built by an Austrian missionary in the late 1970's. During the war in the 1980's, the church was forced to abandon the house. In the 1990's, a general rented it for a few years then stopped paying rent. Since, it's been squatted on by various members of his family.

The Mission wants it back.

The house is on the main road, the only paved road in Moundou. But it's not directly next to the pavement. A soccer field owned by the military base across the street separates the house from the asphalt.

The house itself is in ruins. The roof is leaking and torn. The ceiling is peeling and falling down. What were large windows are now bricked up. Dirt and spider webs are everywhere. Bare electrical wires hang out where switches and plugs used to be. However, one can still see traces of the solid Austrian cement work in the foundations and walls.

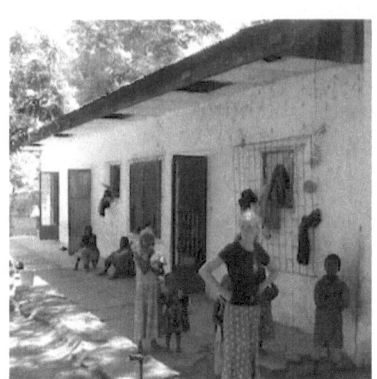

Mission House Moundou

My imagination starts whirling. *If you took out this wall, the back two rooms would make a nice operating room. This room over here could be the minor procedure room as it opens nicely to the veranda. The bathroom could easily become a sterilization room. This living room with large doors on both sides could easily be a pre-op/post-op room. If we walled off the garage we'd have a labor and delivery room. And this front room opening to the outside and to the living room would be a perfect consultation room.*

"Job," I begin. "If we could get the house back, could AHI use it to make a surgery center out of?"

"Of course! That's a great idea. We just want it back in Adventist hands."

We talk to the squatters who have shown us around and they agree to get out at the end of the rainy season in September or October. I go back to Béré with a lot of ideas in my head but no practical plan.

A week later I get an email from the Loma Linda Women's Auxiliary asking if we have any projects that need sponsoring in Tchad. I write back with less than a page describing the project. Before I know it, we have $70,000 for the project! I can't wait to see where this goes!

04 July 2008
Jugular

The dark blood suddenly gushes out of the neck wound like a hot spring bubbling up from the ground...

I had hardly slept the night before anticipating the complexities of operating on this man's neck. He had a mass bulging out under his right mandible which looked like a bunch of large grapes with bearded skin stretched tightly over them. The mass was smooth and lumpy and about the size of a large grapefruit.

He'd been to many other hospitals who'd told him there's nothing that could be done.

The surgery started off bad with a difficult intubation. I put the laryngoscope into his mouth only to find myself faced with a looming open esophagus and no vocal cords in sight. I pulled up with all my strength, tried repositioning the head, had someone try and push his voice box down, all to no avail. Finally, I blindly inserted the tube above where I could see the esophagus and pulled out the guide wire. As my cousin Jenny filled up the cuff with air and my other cousin John attached the Ambu bag, I looked for the telltale signs of vapor on the tube. Then, Jenny verified that there were breath sounds.

Unfortunately, at this time his oxygen saturation started to fall as his pulse jumped up to 172 beats per minute. I listened to his lungs and they were clamped down like a severe asthma attack. I quickly asked Siméon to give him some IV steroids and Chelsey to run to the pharmacy for some bronchodilators.

It was about this time he started to grunt and clench his jaw and hands while straining like he was going to burst through some invisible barrier like the Incredible Hulk transforming himself into the Green Monster. I shouted at Siméon who quickly gave him more Diazepam on top of the Ketamine.

Finally, after about 30 minutes, we had him sedated enough, airway open enough and heart rate down enough to start the hard part of the case.

I had dissected the skin off the mass and was working my way around the lateral side underneath the tumor when I got into the jugular vein...

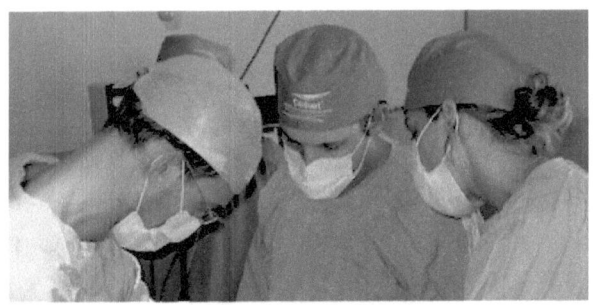

James, John & Jenny

As the blood gurgles into the wound I quickly put my finger over it with a gauze pad between me and the large vein carrying most of the blood from the head. I pause for a moment. What do I do now? I'm definitely in uncharted territory. I calmly ask John to put on some sterile gloves and hold pressure on the wound. As he holds the man's lifeblood from escaping under his finger I continue to methodically and painstakingly dissect the rest of the mass off the mandible, the voice box, the trachea and the carotid artery and other deep muscular neck structures. An hour later, the mass is out.

Johns fingers are paralyzed in position and totally numb. I ask him to gently take off pressure. Blood surges into the surgical field. He quickly presses back down.

It's then I remember my old friend, Erling Oksenholt pulling me into his office in Oregon in May and showing me a short video. In the video, a gloved hand is poised over a pig's groin. A sharp scalpel suddenly lunges down slicing through the porker's femoral artery. As blood spews from the wound the gloved hand quickly piles on gauze and holds down fiercely. Then, just as quickly, the gauze is withdrawn and a white powder is poured into the wound and the gauze and pressure is quickly reapplied. A note on the bottom of the screen says "five minutes later" as the scene shifts slightly. The gloved hand releases pressure and gently pulls up the gauze. There is no bleeding.

I also remember that Erling gave me some packets of this miracle powder (Celox) that I had left with my cousin John to bring with him when he came three days ago.

I yell to Brian to run over and check the bags that he and John brought and see if he couldn't find any. Meanwhile, John and I continue to wait and hold pressure. Brian comes back at first to say he didn't find any. Jenny and Chelsey go to help him look. Finally, Brian comes back with a small, white plastic bag with Celox written on it in big red letters. Brian opens the sack.

After a few seconds, I say, "Ready!" and lift off the gauze as he quickly pours in the powder and I reapply pressure. Five minutes later I lift off the gauze and see white powder in the wound but no bleeding.

John has been reading the instructions and says that now I should irrigate the powder out of the wound which I do. At the end I am trying to wipe out the last fragments and the blood gushes forth again. We repeat the process and the second time I'm a little gentler.

It holds. I close the muscles and skin. I wrap his head and neck in a loose ace wrap. Then, I send him off to ICU attached to a ventilator—whoops, dreaming again. Instead, I take out his endotracheal tube and send him out to the hot, sticky wards where his family will fan him with homemade woven fans and we'll hope he wakes up and his throat doesn't swell up too much so that he can't breathe.

Two days later he complains of a sore throat but is sitting up, breathing normally and taking liquids. His neck has virtually no swelling at all.

31 July 2008

Eclampsia

Boom! Boom! Boom! The pounding on our cheap, metal front door jolts me out of a deep sleep. I glance quickly at my watch: 4:13 AM.

"James! James! Are you awake?!" I hear Dr. Bond's son, Gabriel, calling me, out of breath.

I pull on some shorts and fumble my way through the darkness out the bedroom door, past the bookshelf on the left, through the curtains covering the exit, out the living room door and onto the porch.

"What's up?" I mumble, trying to clear the cobwebs.

"Doudjé's wife just came in with seizures and we need some Magnesium from the pharmacy." I notice the shadowy form of Dr. Bond behind Gabriel in the moonless night.

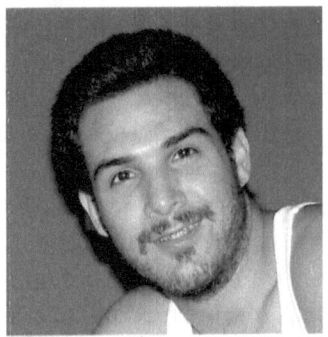

Gabriel

"I'm coming," I reply and head back in to pull on some scrubs, grab my keys and a head lamp and back outside where I hear the voices of Gabriel and Bond fading around the corner of the container across the yard.

I push through the wet leaves of the bushes forming a hedge between our house and Lazare's little hut just outside the main house and stumble over his wire cooking basket. I make my way over to the fence, unlock the gate and head towards the dim light coming from the ER. I hear screams, wails and the sounds of a struggle coming from within that grow louder as I approach at a fast walk.

I push aside the bright green and yellow flowered curtain blocking the entrance to the ER and my eyes are instantly drawn to a group of about ten people surrounding one of the beds. Cries and moans are coming from inside the circle of bodies. A bottle of IV fluids hangs from a wooden IV pole and a tube descends into the crowd. Arms and legs shoot out here and there and are instantly seized by several hands and pushed back inside.

I push the people aside and get my first look. It is certainly Doudjé's wife. She is also Koumakoy and Frederic's sister. I can barely recognize her. I nod to Frederic and his mom who are part of the crowd.

"*Lapia ei?*" I greet them in Nangjéré.

"*Lapia, Jamsuh,*" responds the mom in Nangjéré.

"*Ca va,*" Frederic replies in French.

Doudjé hasn't arrived yet but his wife is swollen up like a balloon with edema everywhere. She is alternating between thrashing and lying moaning on the exam table. Just then she makes a violent effort and pulls out her IV causing blood to splatter all over the bed and floor. A nursing student rushes to stop the bleeding with a cotton ball.

She seems to vaguely recognize me as she looks at me—or more like through me—and mumbles *"Jamsuh, Jamsuh, Jamsuh!"* over and over again.

Augustin, the night nurse, informs me that she came in convulsing with a blood pressure of 140/90. No question about it, it's eclampsia. I had just done an ultrasound on her a few weeks ago and discovered she had twins. There is definitely no time to lose.

"I found both fetal heartbeats," reassures Dr. Bond as I start to bark out orders.

"Augustin, call Siméon and Abel! Gabriel, you and the nursing student go get the gurney and take her to the operating room! David, go call Sarah, tell her we need her immediately! Bond, I'll go get the Magnesium from the pharmacy, here's the keys to the operating room."

We all split as the family continues to hold her down.

I pull out six ampoules of Magnesium and meet the gurney in the operating room just in time to see the next seizure.

As she rolls through the door her body stiffens, her eyes roll back in her head and then she starts shaking violently with her teeth clenched. She starts bleeding again from the old IV site. Then, after a few seconds, the seizure stops and she lays unconscious on the gurney.

"Now's our chance. She's unconscious. Let's get her clothes off, get her in the operating room, start an IV and get her ready for surgery," I shout.

Sarah and Abel have both arrived. Between the two of them they quickly start an IV, put in a foley catheter and inject an antibiotic. Abel helps us transfer her to the operating room table.

I sidle up to Bond and ask him quietly if he minds if I do the surgery. Since I've been following her during her pregnancy, she's the wife of a friend of mine and I myself was a twin born by C-section, I request the privilege of doing the life-saving surgery on her. Bond is generous and concedes me the case. We scrub together.

By this time Siméon has arrived and I tell him to prepare one milliliter of Ketamine. Doudjé's wife is still somnolent. Bond and I scrub and don gowns and gloves. Abel has prepared the surgical field and we drape the lower abdomen.

We pause for prayer and then I take up the scalpel. Two slices later and I see the uterus. Bond stretches the peritoneal opening wider as I insert the bladder retractor. I make a small transverse incision and poke through with a hemostat. I then insert the index finger of both hands and pull out and up opening the uterine wound. There is the upper back and neck of a tiny baby. I insert my hand down into the uterus till I find the head and lift it up and into the uterine wound. Bond pushes the top of the uterus and the baby slides into the world with a gasp and a scream.

Here's where things go temporarily wrong. Bond has grabbed the clamps for the umbilical cord and tells me to go for the next baby. I see the bulging amniotic sac and try to break it with my fingers with no success.

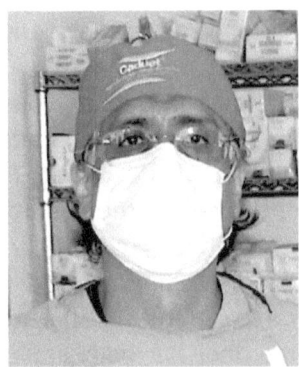

Bond

Then, for some strange reason, I do something I never do, I reach again for the scalpel. As I bring it up to the surgical wound, Bond reaches down to grab some scissors to cut the cord and the scalpel collides with his finger. I'm horrified but Bond signals me to keep going as he finishes cutting the cord and handing off the baby. I put the scalpel down, burst the sac with another instrument and deliver the second baby who also comes out with great tone and grimacing and crying. Bond calls for another glove and we suture closed the uterus, the fascia and the skin with no further complications.

By the end of the surgery, her blood pressure has already normalized. Bond goes off to wash out his wound. We call in the lab to do an HIV test which is negative and Bond starts on post-exposure prophylaxis. By the next day, her edema has started to go down, the twins are breastfeeding. Doudjé is the happiest, proudest man in town. He names his twin boys James and Bond.

11 August 2008
Pins

I feel like an idiot. What was I thinking? Of course, the wound would get infected. I was too optimistic when I wrote that the wound looked great three days later and maybe a miracle would happen. The fracture got infected the next day. I tried to clean it out again and cover the bone with some muscle. That got infected. I tried to cast it in various ways, the bone didn't stay in place and kept pushing out through the wound, seeking the outside air like a drowning man. Nothing seemed to work. I thought maybe we'd have to amputate.

Finally, we just left the whole thing open and let diluted bleach dressings do their trick. Slowly the wound cleaned up and granulation tissue formed. We kept asking if anyone could send us an external fixator. No one could find one. Finally, the wound was clean but the fracture was only partially stabilized and the bone was still exposed.

Sarah just left to go back to Denmark for the next IVF treatment attempt. I wish she were here.

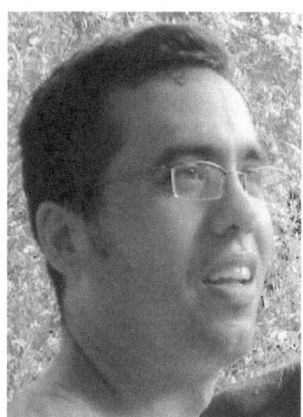

Jason

Fortunately, I have some reinforcements. Dr. Bond and Dr. Jason Shives are with me in Béré. We talk about the open tibia fracture and what to do. Finally, we come up with a brilliant plan straight out of the MacGyver archives. Abel and Siméon prepare the patient while I head over to the house. I find a long piece of two and a half inch pipe that seems pretty strong. I grab a saw from the tool box and cut two pieces off, roughly the length of a certain man's tibia.

Meanwhile, Jason and Abel have brought out the small generator and the cast saw and have been spewing plaster powder all over the ward in an attempt to take of the full leg cast.

We rejoin Bond in the operating room where we try out Bond's regional spinal anesthetic technique by having our patient lie on his left side, the side of the fracture, while we put in the spinal lidocaine and let him sit on that side so only his left leg will be numb. When it's settled in, we turn him back onto his back and I hand the leg off to Gabriel to hold while Abel preps the leg with Betadine.

Jason and I scrub while Bond directs and advises. I first pull out some pieces of infected sequestrum and chip off some of the bone sticking too far out with a rongeur. We twist the leg into a more anatomical position and Gabriel holds it steady.

I follow Bond's suggestion and make four tiny incisions, two above the wound and two below. Then I take a regular, unsterile cordless drill with my right hand and insert a sterile, threaded Steinmann pin into the drill with my still clean left hand. I insert the still sterile end of the pin in one of the incisions and push it against the bone. I then squeeze the trigger and thread the pin in and through the tibia till it pokes the skin on the other side. Jason makes a small cut with the scalpel over the pin and I drill it the rest of the way through till it's sticking out the same amount on both sides. I repeat the processes for the remaining three pins.

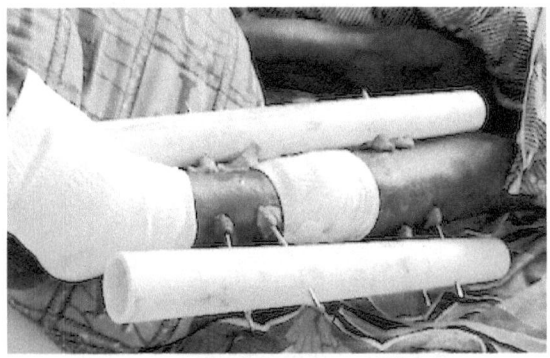

Homemade PVC external fixator

Then, while Jason holds the PVC pipe steady against the pins, I mark where they should go through and then drill holes through the pipe. I then force the pipe over the pins till the pins hit the other side of the pipe. I then try to estimate where I should drill the second holes and mark the pipe again. I drill again and this time get each pin to go through it's second hole with the help of a little hammering. I repeat the process on the other side.

Gabriel lets go his stabilizing hold on the leg and we confirm that the fracture is now stabilized. Jason wraps gauze with Betadine around the pins while I dress the fracture wound with diluted bleach and we take him back out to the ward.

18 August 2008
Futbol

Why did I choose to wear shoes? I thought it would protect my ankle. Last week it was smashed by Jason forming a superficial blood clot. My left inner ankle and foot swelled up and turned different shades of purple and green.

Now as I send the ball skimming back across the grass, in the general direction of where I want it to go, I feel some burning pains on the sides of both small toes.

As Bond, Gabriel, Klevin and Stefan continue to play with some of the neighborhood kids I step behind the two broken bricks marking the goal posts and take off my shoes. Sure enough, blisters have already burst leaving raw flesh where the side of the toes should be.

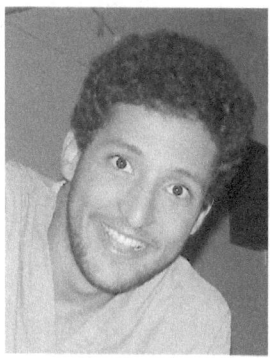

Klevin

I jump back up from the ground and join back in the game. As I look up past the other goal defended so well by Bond things sort of go into movie mode as four well-muscled teenage Tchadians stroll up slowly from past the end of the fence. I almost feel like things should go in slow motion with sinister music from some gang flick plays in the background. The brief moment is burst, however, as they flash large smiles and I recognize Koumakoy and Frederick's brother along with some of the normal neighborhood soccer thugs.

We quickly divide into "us" versus "them." They are intent on preserving the national Tchadian football honor on this warm, Friday afternoon. In fact, warm is an understatement, as the humidity from last night's downpour hangs like a suffocating blanket over the ratty field as a cloudless sky lets a merciless African sun slowly broil us alive.

Needless to say, a few minutes into the match and my scrub bottoms are already soaking with sweat from the waist down and the top has long since been discarded. Klevin, the newly arrived Brazilian medical student and I are the only barefoot ones on our team.

Stefan is our version of a gang banger with his recently shaved head and monstrous sideburns intimidating the opposition almost as much as his bare hairy chest and cleats. Gabriel and Bond also are wearing scrubs and tennis shoes. Our opposition is lean and mean wearing only shorts and the occasional t-shirt along with bare feet or flip flops in various stages of degradation.

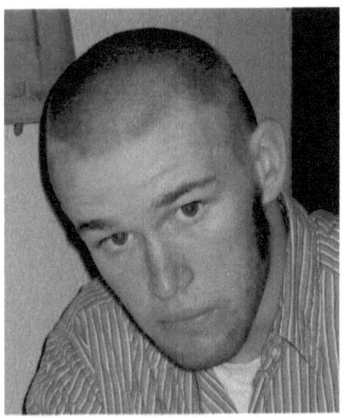

Stefan

We score first. After some footwork only a Brazilian could imagine, Klevin makes a beautiful pass setting up Stefan for a nifty tap in. Second blood is by the Tchadians. A breakdown in passing on my part sets up an easily intercepted ball across the middle and an angle shot off the bricks serving as goalposts. From there on out it's back-and-forth with the Tchadians controlling the ball the majority of the time before losing it through too much dribbling and not enough passing. We on the other hand make the most of our few opportunities and are soon up three to one.

A loud thunder clap from the East makes me look up to see angry clouds forming quickly. They cast a slight shadow over the millet jungle that Béré has become and send a cool breeze across our sweaty bodies. A perfect rainbow encircles the encroaching storm.

As brilliant footwork and sometimes stellar passes continue beneath the now menacing sky, small pellets of water began to drop into the dry dust of the road making up the Western part of our playing field.

I quickly run over and put my Bible and songbook into the open doors of the church just to the Southeast, then grab my shoes and barely get them in before the downpour starts.

But we have not yet begun to play. The game goes on. We are drenched within minutes. Passes start to get sloppy and slow down as the earth turns boggy. The rainbow has disappeared, but there is still clear sky to the West where the sun is almost changing color into sunset. The rain is coming down almost parallel to the ground drilling itself into our burning flesh.

The western part of the field is now almost unplayable. Any pass hazarding into its slimy clutches is instantly stopped in a puddle of water and muddy sand. The Tchadians with flip flops are starting to slip and slide dangerously while the barefooted ones continue with no loss of traction. A huge grin splays across my face as Bond looks on from the eaves of the church having retreated there with the first of the downpour.

I haven't had this much fun in a long time.

Eventually, the Tchadians have had enough. Down five to one I don't blame them. They rub their tummies and give mournful looks as they say they haven't eaten since the morning and have no strength. I mock them comparing our sagging bodies to their chiseled frames, but they just laugh and insist. We finally agree to meet again Sunday and slap hands all around. I head back over to the church as the torrent continues.

The noise inside the tin-roofed church is deafening. The only people who've made it for Friday evening prayer meeting are Lazare and a few kids who come around me as I sit in front of Lazare and say we should sing or something.

Shouting out loudly as we belt out songs in Nangjéré I can tell that the kids are loving it, especially one-armed-boy. Finally after a few rounds of *"Ka Ama Kouma Kwani Teri"* and *"Kela ka dane ma ei kera...dul kang ddi, Jesus, Jesus-Christi"*, I tell them the story of David and Goliath using Lazare to translate from French into Nangjéré.

I end with teaching them the song "Only a Boy Named David" in Nangjéré (*Kware kusi ne David*) by holding the songbook up to the last rays of light coming in the slit that serves as a window on the church. Then, one of the boys prays, Lazare locks up and I walk back slowly home through the mud and the mist.

04 September 2008

Fixin' da bone

Considering I'd only done it once before in my life, it's hard to believe that this is the third time this month I'm slicing open a thigh. This one should be the hardest one to date.

Abel helps me stretch a sticky, yellow plastic covering over the thigh where we'll cut to try and get to the unhealed femur. As I poise with the scalpel over the now yellow window of thigh in the surgical field the first two cases flash through my mind...

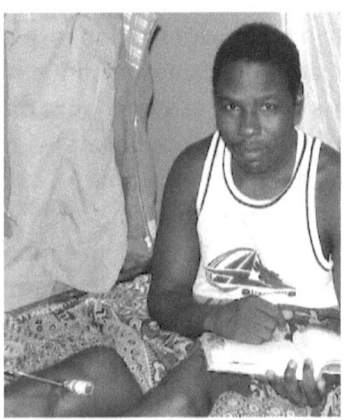

Lamglé

The first was a large man named Lamglé who was hit by a motorcycle two years ago. His twin brother came to our hospital for some other reason. While here, he asked me if I could do anything for his brother whose leg had healed badly after a fracture. He is now crippled hobbling around with the aid of a crutch thanks to his now shortened right leg. Surprisingly, the traditional method of bone setting hadn't worked leaving him with a circumferential scar where they had attached a cord too tightly.

I told him to have Lamglé see me when I'd be in N'Djamena next. Sure enough he showed up with several sets of x-rays showing his femur shortened by four centimeters and angled at about 25 degrees. It was well healed though. When he came to Béré I was able to break the two fragments apart and then put him in traction to pull it out to length. He's been here for a month now.

The second was an eight year old girl named Ma Joie. She was referred by the first patient. In fact, she was his niece or something. She also had a right femur fracture which was three months' old. A motorcycle hit her. I did basically the same procedure on her. She's been here for a couple weeks now. Her hospital stay has been complicated with malaria and anemia needing a blood transfusion. She is stoic and looks me directly in the eyes every time I do rounds. She lifts out her hand solemnly for the obligatory greeting and exchange of "*Ça va? Oui, ça va.*" I look forward to seeing her every day.

I slice through the yellow plastic. The black skin and light yellow fat turn quickly red with blood. I think again that this one won't be as easy...

Another call came to me while I was in N'Djamena last week. A man's voice introduces himself as Mahamat. He tells me that he had heard that we'd operated successfully on two of his relatives with right femur fractures. He hoped we could do the same for him. He has the same problem: a right femur broken by a motorcycle hitting him while he was riding a bicycle.

He brought me his x-rays. As I held them up in the faint rays of light filtering through the slats of the ER windows I could tell instantly that this was more complicated. The two fragments of the femur were separated by about 4-5 cms with a separate fragment also to the side. There was no evidence of any type of callous or new bone formation anywhere.

It was a year already since the accident. His fracture had been an open fracture with a draining wound for three months before it closed. As I looked again at the thigh I saw the healed scars from where the bone shard had pierced the skin. As I picked up his leg I found he had an extra joint mid-thigh. I could move his lower leg in all four directions without his hip moving at all. Not good!

I cut through the fascia and the red muscle wells up into the wound as Abel retracts. As I continue down through the muscle, I see the fibers twitch and retract. I hit some nice arteries and scramble to clamp them off. I call for a suture and tie off the bleeders. I can feel the proximal fragment of bone with a muscle spilling over it down into a cavity where the other bone has to be somewhere.

I keep digging until I find the distal part of the femur. There is about two inches of muscle and a ton of scar tissue all around. I try to free it up with various instruments: scalpel, scissors, periosteal elevators and various others. I get into part of the scar tissue that has walled off some yellow inflammatory liquid like a cyst. It is clear though and happily doesn't look infected. The distal part just doesn't want come free.

I'm kind of a little nervous as I know somewhere around the back or medial side of that deep bone are the big artery and vein that supply the leg. I don't want to have to resort to a Celox miracle again.

I have the scar tissue freed up superiorly, medially and laterally, but behind the bone I just can't seem to get to it. Finally, I find some dangerous looking pincher-like instrument and manage to grasp the fragment and pull it up enough to cut off the scar tissue keeping it from moving.

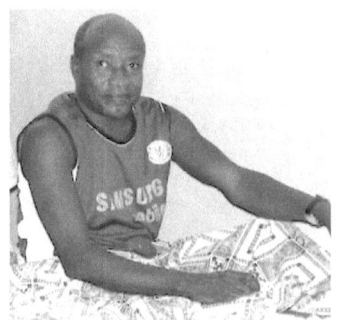

Mahamat

I then grab a rongeur and start ripping, tearing, biting and cracking off pieces of calloused bone over the two unhealed ends. Finally, I'm down to pretty fresh, raw, bleeding bone. Klevin and Gabriel have been taking turns putting some traction on the foot and now I really have them tug with all they've got. The bones are still overlapped by a centimeter. I wedge in a chisel and with my prying and the boys' pulling, the distal part finally slips over the proximal and meshes together with all the sharp edges left after my gnawing at them.

As Klevin and Gabrielle maintain tension on the leg I suture closed the fascias and the skin and place a sterile dressing. I then take out a sterile, threaded pin about 20cm long and put one end into a very not sterile cordless drill. I make a small incision on the skin over the tibia and pull the trigger. The pin barely moves, the battery is weak. It makes it a few millimeters into the bone before conking out completely.

I ask for the other battery. It is also dead since the charger hasn't been plugged in. I try an old rusty hand drill. Doesn't move at all. Finally, I send Gabrielle to my house to get another cordless drill. After a long five minutes he's back. I drill through the bone, nick the skin on the other side and let the pin work it's way halfway through before detaching the drill. I then attach a U-shaped wire onto it so we can attach a bag of sand to work as traction to keep the leg out to length.

We transfer Mahamat from the operating room to his bed. After attaching the sand bag, I perform the final maneuver. I put two empty Ceftriaxone vials over the sharp edges of the pin, confirm that the legs are the same length and go home.

13 September 2008
Insomnia

I've had a nice relaxing day. First of all, I sleep in, thanks to a sleeping pill. Then, I do an appendectomy. When I come home, I watch "The Gospel of John" on DVD, play the guitar, cook some beans and rice, and feed the horses. In the evening, I attend a prayer meeting. Afterwards, I read "Le Comte de Monte Cristo" until 10:00pm when my eyes are so heavy I know I'll fall asleep immediately.

Or so it seems at first. My earplugs seem to drown out all noise. The bed feels very comfortable. It's not too hot. I feel myself sinking into the bed and a deep sleep. But then, slowly, the ear plugs unplug a little. The sounds of children's squeals and shouts breaks through. Drum beats waft over the light of a full moon. I start to feel a little cold. I pull on the sheets. Then my muscles feel a little stiff. I stretch them out. I start to toss and turn. Then I feel hot and take the sheets off. My thoughts start to pour in on themselves...

Maybe I should've taken out that inflamed Cecum instead of just draining the peri-appendiceal abscess. I'll probably have to operate tomorrow. It'll be complicated. Who knows what will happen?

Is that a knock on the door? I pull out my earplugs. Nothing. Then, I hear a faint tapping of knuckles on sheet metal. I pull off the eye shade and the other ear plug. I fumble for some shorts and stumble out to the door. The way is lit by the incandescent blue of the bug lamp. It's Samedi.

"The young man with the snake bite. His dad wants to take him home. I told him he can't be released without the doctor's orders. I tried to convince him to wait until the morning, but he says that everyone in the neighborhood is saying that his son is dead, so he wants to take him home."

"What kind of excuse is that?" I think to myself then reply to Samedi. "Have him sign the form that he's leaving against medical advice. We're not a prison, we can't force anyone to stay. The dad doesn't even care that his son is better. If he was going to die he would've done it the first day or two."

"I've tried to reason with him," Samedi replies. "Even Pierre and Henri tried to talk to him. He's totally beyond reason."

"Ok, *bon travail!*"

I return to my bed and hope that now I'll be able to sleep.

At first, I think it'll work. But then thoughts start to trickle in. Unwanted worries crowd my head. The kids' voices keep penetrating the silence of my ear plugs. Medical and surgical cases keep parading through my subconscious along with preoccupations that I should have done things differently or maybe I should've done this and not done that.

Then, I start thinking about the projects I want to do, all the preventative measures that could be taken...

What are we going to do about malaria? Will DDT spraying ever happen? What about the TB and AIDS patients? Will I ever get time to train the village health care workers like I want to? How are the volunteers going to work out? Am I giving them enough direction? Am I being too controlling?

And what about the Moundou project? I can't believe I've taken on another project. But it just seemed right: Job taking me to see the old mission house being squatted on by the military, my imagining how it could be turned into a surgery center, the Loma Linda Women's Auxiliary giving us $70,000 for the project, finding a good honest builder in Frederic, etc. But it's just added a load to my worries...

As I fitfully fall into a light slumber, the tossing and turning continues. Just as I seem to be asleep I wake up, my heart beating fast having dreamt once again that I'm having to flee something, that I need to escape, something that is chasing me and almost finds me. Every time, though, they miraculously overlook my obvious hiding place. It's a recurrent nightmare.

Is that a knock on the door? I pull out the right earplug.

"*Oui?*" I ask. I look out the small bedroom window onto the porch. The moon illuminates the door. There's no one there.

I'm cold again. Now I'm hot. Oh, it's so comfortable on my back as I stretch my legs out. Now it's uncomfortable. Maybe on my side. I should've taken another sleeping pill.

I pull out my earplugs. The dancing and singing and playing has stopped. The crickets and frogs are blasting a cacophony around the house. Somewhere a rooster crows. His friends answer from all over the neighborhood. A tint of red lights up the windows. Dawn is on it's way.

14 September 2008
Shocking

I stand at the foot of her bed. Kristin and Augustin are the nurses on duty and the three nursing students, Ndilbé, Honoré and Innocent are gathered around, white coats spotless, notebooks and charts in hand.

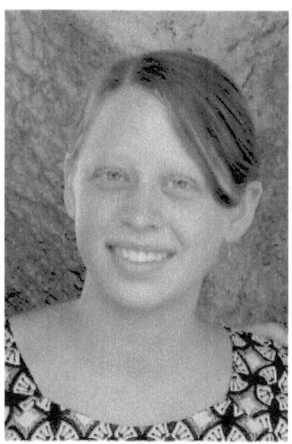

Kristin

The patient has just come out of surgery two days ago for a walled off, perforated appendicitis. At first glance, she seems to be doing fine. She's staring at me with understanding eyes and breathing rapidly but easily. Then, I notice beads of sweat all over her chest, face and arms. I pull off my stethoscope from around my neck and press it against her thorax. The heart beat is rapid and irregular. She's mid thirties and shouldn't have heart disease. What is it?

I look at the chart. Her vital signs there are listed as normal. Then I notice that she's been still kept NPO (nothing to eat or drink) but hasn't got IV fluids in 24 hours. I quickly have the nurse put up some Ringer's lactate IV solution. I think maybe she's dehydrated and has some electrolyte imbalances. We can now at least check her potassium thanks to a donation from Denmark. I go ahead and give her a little expired Magnesium that I've been hording in a little stash in the pharmacy.

Then, I remember the heart monitor-defibrillators that our two young volunteers for the summer brought over. I go to the operating room stock room and find one that still has a charged battery despite never being charged since arrival in Tchad three months ago.

I hook it up to the patient. The screen is so small and the heart beat so fast it's hard to tell for sure, but it looks like atrial fibrillation or atrial flutter. She's gotten a couple liters of fluid and the magnesium. Now the potassium level comes back normal. She seems stable enough so I leave the monitor hooked up but turn it off to save battery. We move on to the next patient. Maybe she'll come out of it on her own.

It's 9:30am.

After finishing rounds and seeing the first batch of ER patients I perform a hernia operation using mosquito net mesh. Then I go to my office to do some ultrasounds.

Augustin knocks on the door. "*Ça ne va pas*," he says. "Bed 10 is in respiratory distress."

I hurry over to the ward, worried that she's already dead. "*Ça ne va pas*" coming out of a nurse's mouth usually means cardiopulmonary arrest. Fortunately, not only is she still alive, but she's conscious and not really in respiratory distress. However, as I turn on the monitor, I see that her heart beat is still 150-160 and irregular. I feel I should do something but it's been a long time since I've had to deal with cardiac patients. I'm not exactly in the best equipped place to deal with it either.

I hurry back my office to look up my little cheat sheet on electrical cardioversion. It tells me I should sedate the patient first if possible, put the defibrillator on sync-mode and start with 100J. Ok, I feel a little better, it's starting to come back.

I hook up the defibrillator pads, give her some Valium, turn on sync-mode and see the little dots appear over the QRS complexes on the EKG. I turn the knob to 100J and hit charge. I hear the whirring of the charge and then it's ready. But now, I don't know how to make it discharge. I look all over and see nothing. Great.

I turn everything off, remove the pads and return to the operating room where I find the paddles with their large, curlycue phone cable-like cords. I hook them into the defibrillator, check out the little buttons and place one over her sternum and the other on her left side under her armpit.

"Everyone back," I announce. "Don't touch the bed or anything!"

She's still staring up at me wondering what the heck I'm doing. But then again, I'm wondering the same thing! I see that the QRS complexes are synced. I hit the charge button and then the two shock buttons. Just like in the movies or on TV she bounces a little off the bed, her head flies back, and then she flops back down. The EKG makes a big waveform, a brief flat-line and then a normal rhythm of 110 beats per minute starts to play across the little green screen.

I almost can't believe it. I know it's supposed to work according to all I've read and been told in my ACLS courses. But come to think of it, even in the USA I don't think I've ever been present for a synchronized cardioversion.

My heart is full with thanks to God for bringing everything together to make it possible for us to save this woman's life first with the operation and then with what I had considered mostly useless defibrillator monitors.

Shocking!

26 September 2008
Road-trip

"I don't know," I say to Sarah on the phone. "I really want to pick you up in the airport, but it'd be hard now. It's pouring down rain. The roads are already bad. The car doesn't start. I'd have to go by motorcycle and public transport. I'd like to see you as soon as possible, but I'm exhausted. Plus the extra expense...couldn't you just take a taxi from the airport and then come down on public transport?"

Sarah has been in Denmark for a month for some infertility treatments. We did IVF earlier in the year, but it didn't work. However, we had some embryos that were frozen so Sarah has gone to do another cycle. She's is supposed to arrive tomorrow in N'Djamena. She may or may not be pregnant. However, travel is so difficult during the rainy season...I try to excuse myself. Deep down, I feel I should go to meet her, but she doesn't have to know that!

I haven't decided for sure one way or another, but I get a text message from her later that evening. She tells me that she understands and I should feel free to not come to pick her up. I'll just owe her a ton of back rubs later!

I call Ndilbé, a nursing student who has just finished his three month internship and is ready to go back to N'Djamena.

"I'd like to travel with you to N'Djamena," I say. "Can we leave tomorrow at 5:00am?"

Ndilbé nods.

"Can you arrange some *motos* for us then?" I ask.

He nods again.

At 3:00am, Augustin knocks on my door. "There's a kid in respiratory distress, can you come see him."

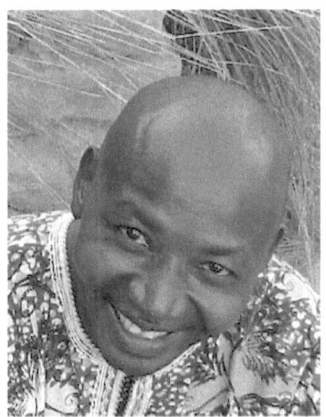

Augustin

"Sure," I reply. I haven't been able to sleep anyway thinking about surprising my wife at the airport.

The kid is grunting, wheezing, retracting and has nasal flaring. Severe asthma. I open my office and find a few vials of expired Xopenex that we put in the nebulizer. I tell Augustin to give him some Dexamethazone IM while I hook up the machine.

The kid suddenly comes alive and starts thrashing around. It's all the mom and I can do to hold him close enough to the mask for some of the medication to get in his lungs. Despite his best efforts, something must be getting in those tiny lungs since he starts to breath easier. I tell Augustin to start a Quinine drip for malaria and Ampicillin in case it's pneumonia that triggered the attack. I return home.

I'm too wired to go back to sleep. I make some egg gravy and toast for breakfast. I finish packing my small backpack. I put in a skirt and t-shirt for Sarah along with an army duffle bag so she can bring back fresh vegetables from the N'Djamena market.

The predawn glow appears. It's cool yet humid. A haze rests across the African plain. Two old Nigerian motorcycles with dim headlights waxing and waning with the speed of the engine limp up to the front gate spewing out white, burned-oil-smelling exhaust. One of them already carries Ndilbé. As I mount my ride, Ndilbé wraps himself up in a turban. We strap our bags to the back of the *motos* with old bicycle inner tubes.

And we're off, with the cool air whipping gritty humidity into our faces. The road is one long series of mud puddles with improvised footpaths around most of them extending sometimes into the rice fields. Often we have to plow through green, muddy water midway up the tires.

We cross the new bridge and down the other side where the gravel buttress has almost completely fallen away. The rains have eroded most of it leaving just a small middle section held together with a few beams and cables haphazardly holding things together. We pass the security check point at the bottom and continue through Tchoua on our way to the lake where the hippos hang out.

The elevated road through the lake has a central drainage pipe. The surface is pock marked with a million ruts carved out by heavy trucks and a billion ridges carved out by the draining rainwater. The rains have turned the clay slick making it a bumpy slip and slide experience. I can't help but wonder when we'll just slide down into that wide open hippo mouth.

The last stretch before Kélo is completely submerged. We plow our way through. The muddy streets of Kélo are lined with tiny mud brick shops just yawning a good morning to another day of fasting in this month of Ramadan. A few lonely robed figures stroll through the red tinged early morning fog. We finally hit the pavement and pull up to the "bus station". On the opposite side of the road I see an air compressor and rickety wooden tables lined with various shapes and sizes of glass bottles filled with an assorted variety and mixture of fuels.

After paying the *moto* taxi-men, we buy our bus tickets. A young, turbaned man approaches and greets us. He is chewing on the typical Muslim teeth cleaning stick. It's the son of the businessman building our new junior high in Béré. He's on his way to Cameroon to study. I buy some bananas and then confirm he's fasting by offering him one which he politely refuses.

We get on the bus and have two of the back four seats. Ndilbé takes one window and I take the other. Next to Ndilbé is another robed, turbaned Muslim. He occasionally spits out the window to keep from violating one of the Five Pillars by inadvertently swallowing his saliva. A fully covered and veiled Muslim woman with dark gloves and stockings makes her way down the aisle towards the back. A young Arab in front of me seems concerned that this obviously pious woman may be forced to sit by an obviously foreign—and thus necessarily infidel—white man. He shouts in Arabic to Ndilbé and the other man to move over which they do.

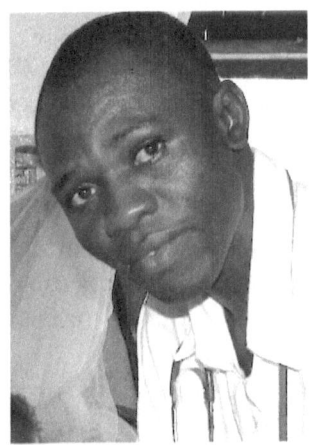

Ndilbé

"*Da bas adil,*" he nods his approval as the deeply perfumed, modest example of virtue makes her way to the seat as far away from me as possible in the same row on a tiny bus. I'm relieved too.

I pass the rest of the four hour trip reading a "Tale of Two Cities" and napping occasionally. We arrive without incident in the midst of a busy market in N'Djamena.

I had planned to catch a taxi straight to the mission guest house, but decide to go with Ndilbé instead. We need to go pay his nursing school fees for the next academic year.

We walk down the crowded, noisy market street and turn the corner. We hail a small Peugeot taxi, but as we're putting our bags in the back, three people have got in the back seat and two in the front. There's only one space left. We start arguing with the passengers. We have to travel together since I don't know how to get to Ndilbé's place. The woman in the back who'd stolen my spot doesn't budge and just sits there with a smirk on her face. Finally, a young Muslim girl is kind enough to get out of the front seat. I cram myself next to a very large woman occupying the other half of the tiny passenger seat.

The trip is short. Off the main road, we take another street with a drainage ditch in the middle. In the ditch, several small, bare-footed boys search for something in the muck.

We open the gate to the house where Ndilbé is living and enter the courtyard. We dump our bags under a shade tree. I'm thankful to find a latrine in the corner and empty a very full bladder.

The house belong's to Aimé, one of Tchad's chief justices and a member of the Adventist Health International country board. His wife, Neloumta, greets us and generously lets me use her car. We are soon on a bumpy ride through the suburbs of N'Djamena. Fifteen minutes later we arrive at a three story structure. Two secretaries sit doing their nails and gossiping in front of empty administration offices. The people we need to see are out.

"When will they be back?" I ask innocently.

Looking up with an annoyed look, one of the secretaries deigns to reply, "Sometime...maybe tomorrow..."

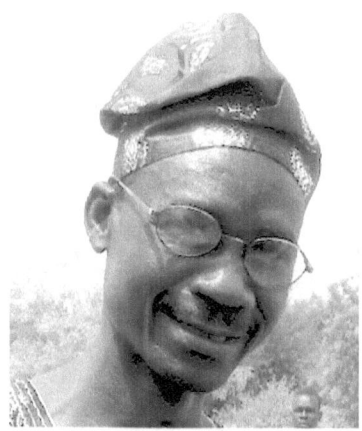

Benzaki

As we leave the school, I get a call from Babana Benzaki who has arrived from Nigeria. A former Muslim originally from Tchad, he converted to Christianity while studying in Nigeria. He is in his last year of public health at Babcock University. Adventist Health International just voted to help him with his school fees for the his final year. After he's finished he'll come work for us for ten years.

Back at Aimé's house, we find Benzaki waiting for us. We sit in the courtyard and converse about health, life and God. In the meantime, Kaitama, the Education Director for the Tchad Adventist Mission, shows up to get the letter I brought from his brother.

Another Adventist Health International board member, Dieudonne Kabdana, stops by on his way home from work. We finalize plans for taking off the lipoma from his neck tomorrow.

Neloumta comes out to the courtyard to invite us in. It's the birthday of her four year old son. With nothing but a couple of boiled eggs and some bananas in my stomach since 4:30am I am more than happy to be part of the celebration! The party ends with some cold Adventist party drinks: dark red hibiscus flower tea and some strong homemade ginger juice.

I finally head to the TEAM guest house in Aimé's Toyota 4-Runner which he's generously let me borrow. I crash for a few hours rest before the 9:00pm arrival of my Danish wife.

At the airport a few hours later, I stand patiently outside the barred entrance to the baggage claim. Various "important" people are let through while others are kept out. Finally, the guards seem to be letting down their vigilance and I slip through with the next batch let in.

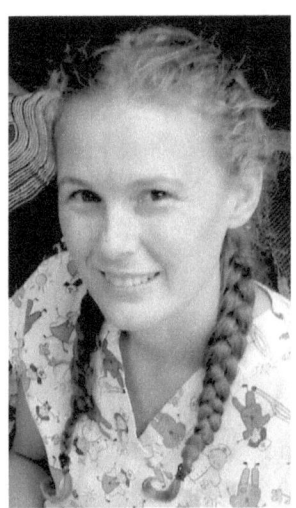

Sarah

I wait in front of the door leading to the immigration booths. I glance in quickly trying to see Sarah's red head without her seeing me. I spot her standing in line. Finally, after a long wait, she appears at the door and looks at me with a shocked look. Then she starts laughing.

"No, no, no, I can't believe it," she spurts out. Unfortunately for me, it's not a pleasant surprise at seeing me that has brought on this reaction. Rather she is shocked at seeing my recently smoothly shaven scalp. She is very cute with her long red hair pulled up in back with a few ringlets of curls escaping to the sides to run down her cheeks and forehead. I give her a warm hug and breath in the fresh smell of her hair as I kiss her head. It's good to have her back!

29 September 2008
Police

I take Sarah and our new Danish volunteer, Nathaniel, to the central market. I'm still in the Toyota 4-Runner I borrowed from Aimé. I park right in front of the Grand Mosque, just ahead of where the taxis pick up and let off passengers. I roll down the windows and sit back to watch the passersby.

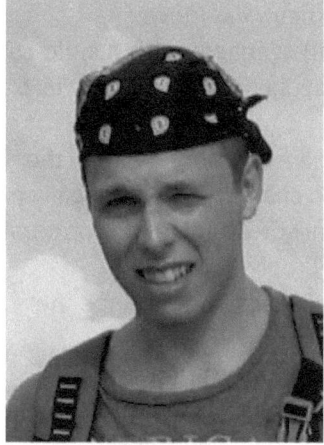

Nathaniel

A few kids come up with their metal bowls asking for alms for the mosque. I chat a little with them in my broken Arabic. One sticks his hand in and is fascinated by seeing the locks go up and down with just the push of a button. Finally, I can't get rid of them, even with the usual "*Allah eftah*" (God will provide) which should be followed by an "*Amin*" and a quick departure. Instead these kids just say "*Ma fi*" (no way). Finally, I grab a bowl, toss it to the side and glare at them. They get the hint.

A young, beak-nosed Arab greets me from behind on the left. I turn my head and greet him back. As I turn back, I see Sarah coming up to the window. She's just finished changing money and is about to head out to buy vegetables.

"Who was that guy and what was he doing by the window?" she asks.

"Nothing, he was just saying hi."

"Oh, he just looked suspicious."

"Don't worry about it. See you in a bit."

She heads out again accompanied by Nathaniel carrying a green army duffle bag.

A brand-new dark green pick up approaches from the left. "*Police*" is written in bold letters across the door. There are machine gun toting gendarmes in the back. A man wearing camouflage with a maroon beret sticks his head out the passenger window, spots me, turns back and says something in Arabic. I hear the word "*Nasara*" and the truck pulls in just in front of me and parks.

Oh boy here we go again.

Sure enough, the man with the beret and several others carrying AK47s hop out and approach the right side of the 4-Runner. I'm a bit surprised, however, by their next move.

A young, gap-toothed teenager with his old school Russian automatic weapon opens the passenger door and gets in beside me, his gun slung loosely by his left side.

"Let's go to the police station!" barks the beret-wearing man, in French. He's obviously in charge. "You're illegally parked."

For some reason I'm not afraid, just exasperated. I try not to sound angry and frustrated as I reply.

"I didn't know I was illegally parked since there is no sign and I've seen others park here before."

The chief doesn't budge. I try a new tactic.

"I can't go because my wife is in the market and how will she know where I've gone and how will I find her?" I can see he's not convinced. "Thanks for informing me that I can't park here. I'll just move the car. Tell me where I can park and thanks for the warning, I won't park here again."

"You can park there on the other side."

I start up the car, back up and cross the one-way traffic to the other side, right in front of the mosque. It seems to me this is a more likely spot to have a no parking sign, but I keep this thought to myself.

My passenger is still with me grinning stupidly at me from time to time as he caresses his weapon. The head honcho follows us over on foot.

"Well, now that you've told us about *Madame*," he begins the negotiations. "We'll let you off easy this time with just a 6000 CFA fine."

I then pull out what I think is my ace. I reach into the glove compartment and pull out an invitation signed by the president of the republic to the year end meeting of the Supreme Court.

"This isn't even my car," I suggest. "Do you really want to haul off one of the supreme court justice's cars? One who's intimate with the Head of State himself?"

"Well, you're the one driving it now!" he retorts. "So it's you who gets to pay the fine."

Touché. At this point, a young man approaches me from the left with a bag of something.

"Are you Dr. James from Béré?" he asks.

"Yes," I reply, grateful for the distraction. Wasting the other person's time is an important element of the bargaining process.

"I've been looking all over for you. I'm the son of the man with the broken femur you operated on last week. I tried to find you earlier at the Mission guest house but I was told you weren't there. Then, my dad told me you were at the National Security Counsel office but I barely missed you there too."

"Yeah, I was there registering our new volunteer for the hospital. He just came back from Denmark with my wife. I called your dad back and told him to have you meet me here."

"So what's up with the *gendarmes*?" he inquires.

I explain the situation to him. He goes to the chief and starts explaining.

"*Chef*, this man is new in town and doesn't know the rules. *Pardon.* He's the head doctor from the Béré Hospital. He just operated on my dad who's also a *policier, s'il vous plaît...*

The chief officer seems to be convinced...a little. He turns to me.

"Well, since you didn't really know...and since you're here helping us out...we'll only make you pay 3000 CFA."

My new friend has now gone over to the other side to talk more intimately with the police. He starts off in French but the officer quickly switches to Arabic saying he doesn't want me to hear their negotiations. Unfortunately for him, I now understand a little Arabic and reply in Arabic that I understand him fine, thank you very much for asking.

He looks at me surprised and starts to laugh good-naturedly.

"Well, you obviously have money since you're driving a car so just share some with us for our tea."

"*Gurus ma fi*," I respond in Arabic. "If I did have money, why would I come from Béré on *motos* and public transport?"

The young gendarme next to me now has a huge gap-toothed grin. He shakes his finger at me in wonder "*Inta da, inta da*...You...you..." and gets out. They all walk off shaking there heads and laughing. Right before getting into their truck they turn one last time and offer a friendly wave goodbye.

As I thank my new friend and offer to carry the sack of homemade pasta to his convalescing dad in Béré, Sarah returns with Nathaniel.

It's then I realize that my cell phone has been stolen. In talking more with Sarah, it seems the guy she saw earlier and asked me about must have been the thief. He was on the right side of the car and was just pulling his head out of the window when she saw him. I thought she was talking about the guy on my left. Apparently, that guy was the thief's partner. He greeted me from behind on the left to distract me long enough for his partner in crime to reach in the open window and take the cell phone from the central console. A slick maneuver I must admit.

05 October 2008

Le week-end

It is still dark and sticky when I wake up around 4:00am thanks to the pitter patter of little rat feet running back and forth directly over my head. Now, I can't go back to sleep. Every time I'm about to find dreamland again I hear the scurrying of the mice or the flapping of a bat outside my screen window. I give up and get out of bed.

I put on a headlamp, trying not to wake Sarah, and go out to the kitchen table. I grab my French Bible and finish preparing the sermon I'll give in church later on this morning. At 5:00am I'm finally able to catch a few more winks. Then the pink early morning light filters in the windows accompanied by the crowing of the ever vigilant roosters.

I eat a simple breakfast of toast with peanut butter and guava sauce. Meanwhile, Sarah has gone out to feed the horses and locked me in! I stare out the bedroom window waiting for someone to come within calling range. Kitty hops up to the window sill to join me in my quiet contemplation of the African dawn. Some purple, pipe-cleaner type flowers have shot up just outside the screen and a bee striped like a zebra is buzzing merrily among the bristles. Everything is green. The guavas are getting bigger and bigger, although they're still not ripe.

Finally, I spot Emily, a volunteer who just arrived yesterday. She responds to my pleas for freedom and unbolts the outside latch on the front door. I pack up my books in a tiny bag, hoist my heavy, hollowed-out-tree-trunk drum to my shoulder and head off to the church.

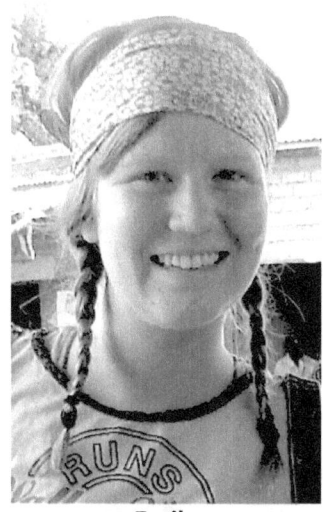

Emily

The sound of French hymns sung off key comes wafting out of the church. As soon as I'm inside, Augustin's son Allah helps produce a more African rendering by pounding out some rhythms on my drum. I accompany him on my little tambourine.

A bit later during the study time, I have a very interesting discussion with a bunch of young people interested in finding out what Christianity is about. We talk about the Bible, how it came about and who wrote it. We talk about the fact that it's a collection of stories telling us how God interacts with people despite all their warts and wrinkles.

Towards the end of the church service, I preach my sermon in French while Doudjé translates into Nangjéré. Afterwards, Siméon is waiting for me outside the church.

"There are a couple of patients you should come see."

I hurry home, change into scrubs and mosey off to the hospital.

Polycarpe, the child with the bleeding disorder we've been transfusing almost every week for the last few months, is having severe abdominal pain. He also had some bloody diarrhea. I'd been saving the plasma part of other people's blood transfusions by storing them in the kerosene freezer. Yesterday, the nurses were supposed to thaw it out, let any remaining red blood cells filter out and give Polycarpe the plasma. It hasn't been done. I quickly hook him up to the plasma and give him some malaria medication. I hope to avoid another transfusion.

A three year old child with a hemoglobin of 4.3 still hasn't got a blood transfusion. Seven family members have been tested but no one has compatible blood. Her blood type is B-, the same as mine. I just gave blood last week, but I have enough to spare. I tell Siméon to call the lab tech, find IV access on the kid and when they're ready I'll donate a pint.

I figure I'd better eat something first, so I go home. Sarah has heated up yesterday's eggplant spaghetti sauce. We eat and then I drink a liter of water and head back to the hospital.

Mathieu is waiting for me. I lie down on the examining table in my office. Mathieu prepares the blood bag, wraps a tourniquet around my arm, uses alcohol soaked cotton to wipe off the skin over the big vein in the middle of my antecubital fossa and slides in a huge needle effortlessly. I pump my fist to make the blood go out faster and quickly fill up the 450ml bag. Mathieu takes out the needle and puts a cotton ball over the puncture wound. I fold my arm, sit up and get ready to go.

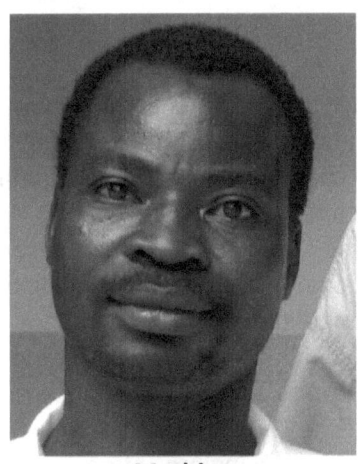

Mathieu

"*Déjà?*" Mathieu asks, astonished. "Aren't you dizzy?"

"*Non*, I just ate and drank a bunch. *Ça va.*"

I head out the door and meet Sarah at the house. She's already saddled Bob. Sarah takes off on Pepper, while the volunteers follow on foot. I change into jeans, grab some water bottles and jump on Bob. Allah is waiting for me so he can get a ride. I swing him up by his arm into the saddle behind me. We take off at a trot. Allah can't keep rhythm with the horse and bounces a lot. We have to stop and walk often, but eventually we catch up to the others.

The rice fields are completely swamped. The path is nothing but a swath of still water meandering among the rice stalks which are already starting to bend at the neck from the weight of their kernels.

It's blazing hot and the water splashing up from Bob's hooves is a welcome, if mild, relief from the sweltering heat.

The river has overflown it's banks swallowing up all the familiar landmarks except a few trees bravely sticking their branches up from the swirling eddies. I dismount and wade out towards the current through what used to be a large field leading down to the cattle crossing. Jason, Jacob and Nathaniel have already almost reached the current as I start out. They are quickly swept downstream. I find the current and swiftly catch up to them where they rest holding onto some branches sticking out of the water. The water rushing by makes it sound like we're in a mountain stream rather than a flat river winding through the African bush.

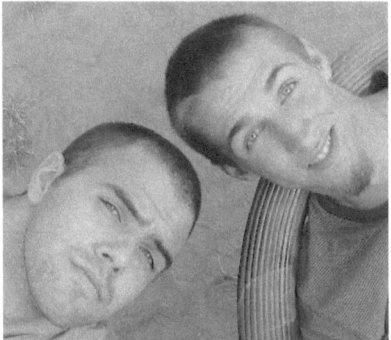

Jacob & Jason

I'm vaguely scared of hippos, though they probably won't like the fast current. I am glad there are no crocs in these rivers.

After several bends we pull ourselves up the bank by grabbing onto piles of tall grasses. We follow the sketchy, overgrown paths through the bush on the bank of the river trying to be as loud as possible to scare off vipers. Back at the ford, Sarah and the others are playing with some of the Tchadian kids. The guys and I head up river where we see a tree coming out of the river near the bank. It bends out conveniently at a perfect angle for jumping.

Jacob hops in feet first to test the depth. It's plenty deep so we dive and do back flips venturing ever higher on the thinner branches until we've exhausted all the possibilities.

Heading home I have a hard time holding Bob back. He smells his supper of dried corn already! Packs of mosquitoes buzz along with us in the twilight as the sun has gone down over half an hour ago. Finally, Allah can't take any more so once we hit the first huts of the village he climbs off. I let Bob go and we gallop off through the approaching night. The wind rushes past leaving the mosquitoes far behind.

I arrive at the compound just in time to see Augustin returning from church. He informs me that Samedi is looking for me. There was a motorcycle accident with some casualties.

I quickly pull off Bob's muddy saddle and harness and put them in the shed. I go home, strip off my soaked jeans, take a fast shower and pull on scrubs. I head over to the hospital.

The ER is dimly lit by one fluorescent bulb buzzing with insects. A small pool of blood is forming at the foot of one bed. A portly, middle-aged woman lies with her left ankle at an impossible angle. A blood-soaked gauze pad is tied on tightly over the wound. I assume it's an open fracture. She has no other injuries.

Another group has just brought in another elderly woman in a push cart. I can tell she needs an amputation just by the smell. Her left foot is wrapped in dirty rags over a mud soaked gauze bandage. I take some scissors and cut off the dressing. Her toes are black and moist: wet gangrene. The calloused skin on the sole is peeling off. A large wound on top reveals tendons and bones mixed with puddles of pus.

A man with a swollen hand is introduced as the motorcycle driver who ran over the woman. He probably has some broken metacarpals. Both women need surgery. The family members discuss among themselves. As I wait, I apply a cast to the man's hand and wrist. I give him some Ibuprofen and tell him to go to Moundou for x-rays.

The family of the woman with the broken ankle are having internal conflicts. No one wants to be financially responsible. Meanwhile, the son of the woman with the rotten foot has paid half of the fees. For the rest, he's signed over his bicycle on as collateral. I'll do her surgery first.

I hope to only have to do a mid-foot amputation. I squeeze the blood out of her leg with an elastic bandage, apply a blood pressure cuff as a tourniquet and slice through the bottom of her foot right into a hidden pocket of pus. I won't be able to save her foot. I move up to the middle of the lower leg and slice down to the bone. I elevate the tissue off the bone as far up as I can. I slowly saw through the tibia and fibula. Progress is slow since I only have a tiny, inch-long bone saw. It keeps getting clogged up with wet bone paste. Finally, I get the leg sawed off. I toss it in the trash. I identify the major vascular bundles. I clamp and tie them off. I suture the muscles and skin over the stump.

The second woman has finally found a solution to her financial problem. Siméon finds an IV then gives her some Ketamine and Diazepam. I yank and tug at her foot trying to reduce the fracture. The fibula gets stuck on some tissue inside. Struggling on I manage to free it up. The foot is now in an anatomically normal position. The medial malleolus is crushed into several pieces. The lateral malleolus seems to have only a single fracture, but it's an open. Abel mixes up some diluted bleach solution and I copiously irrigate the wound.

I close the subcutaneous tissues and dress the wound with Betadine-soaked gauze. While I try to hold the foot and ankle in position, Jacob wraps the leg up to the knee with web roll and then applies a plaster cast. The plaster of Paris is malleable and I am able to mold the ankle some more. The cast hardens and Siméon and Abel take her out to the wards.

It's 11:00pm. I go home. I haven't eaten since lunch. In the meantime, I've given blood, rode horseback to the river, swam, jumped off trees, galloped back and done two operations. I'm famished. Going into the kitchen I find a skillet filled with fried rice and eggs. I devour it. Later, Sarah informs me the food was supposed to be tomorrow's breakfast.

I fall fast asleep until the rat wakes me up again. This time he's let me sleep in till 5:30am. Sarah and I get up. We grab some shovels and a pickax and head out behind the church to dig a latrine...

11 October 2008

Cripple

My life as a cripple begins insignificantly enough.

It's early Sunday morning. I'm digging a latrine. I accidentally hit the inside of my right ankle with the pickax. It doesn't cause any apparent damage. I don't give it a second thought. By evening, however, the ankle is swollen and painful. By next morning, I can barely walk and the overlying skin has turned red. I try to go to work. I hobble around on seeing patients until I can't tolerate the pain anymore.

To top it off, I start to feel like I have Malaria. I limp home. By now, my muscles are twitching. I'm shivering and my teeth are chattering so hard my jaws are getting sore.

I swallow all eight of a new, single-dose anti-malarial treatment straight from China. I huddle under several blankets, desperately trying to feel warm even though my skin is burning hot.

And my ankle is more and more tender by the minute.

After a day or two of convalescence, my malaria symptoms are gone. However, by now I haven't walked in almost a week. I've been hoping for no surgical emergencies. I do get called in for two cases of cephalic-pelvic disproportion. I am able to do the needed symphysiotomies resting my bad leg on a rolling stool. It was definitely worth all the discomfort to hear two newborns screaming at the top of their tiny lungs.

Otherwise, things have been relatively calm.

Six days after the injury, I lounge around home on a lazy Saturday afternoon. I elevate my foot to control the edema. I'm listening to a talk about living in the End Times. Around 5:00pm, I feel the urge to look out the window. I pick up my crutches—which I borrowed from a bed-ridden patient—and limp over to the screen door. Facing me is the fence between us and the Emergency Room.

Something is happening. It's hard to see because of the distance. I make out a group of people gathering rapidly. A couple of push carts move back and forth. Two people are carrying someone on a stretcher. A few minutes later, one of our new nurses, Aimée, comes up the path to the house.

"There's a situation," she blurts out, gasping for breath. "There's been a fight at the market. They've brought in a bunch of victims. One woman's dead. A man has a huge knife wound to his neck. This other woman is all beat up around the head and unconscious. There's a baby that's been wounded..."

"Ok, ok," I interrupt. "I'll be right there!"

I pull on scrubs as quickly as a cripple can manage. I cram my swollen foot into my Crocs and hobble over to the hospital. Trying to walk on crutches over moist, sandy soil is not easy.

I pull aside the curtain at the entrance to the ER. Groups of people huddle around. There are bloody clothes everywhere. Arms and legs poke out of bundles of rags. Some patients are on beds, some on the ground. Sarah looks up from where she's been examining a young woman.

"I think this one is the most critical," she states. "She's pregnant. I can't find the fetal heart beat. She has a huge wound on her head."

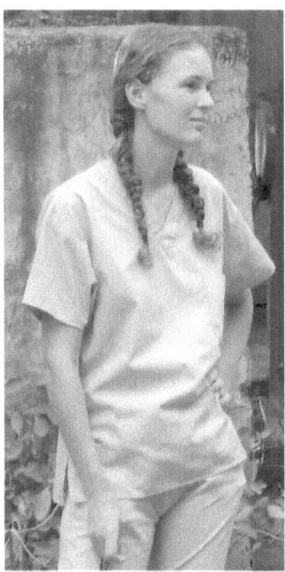

Sarah

In the midst of a bloody pile I see a slender, young Arab girl. Her stomach is bulging, pushing out a brightly colored dress shining with fresh blood. Her swollen face is deformed and bloodied. One eye is completely shut. Her long, tight braids are matted with dark clots.

"One pupil doesn't react well," Jason pipes up, lifting up a light from her eyes. I don't bother to confirm.

Samedi and Abel arrive. Siméon comes shortly thereafter. Ansley, Kristin, Emily and Jacob are also there. I start shouting out orders.

"Get IV's started on everyone. Everyone gets a liter of Ringer's running full speed. Give them all two grams of Ampicillin.

"Where's Stefan? Stefan, get a carton of those one liter Ringer's that just came yesterday.

"Is there a pharmacist? Where's Pierre?"

"I'll call him and get him right in," says André calmly. He's already punching numbers on his cell phone.

"That guy there is probably the second sickest," Sarah shouts across the room as she attaches tubing to the IV on the first patient.

A young man is staring at me calmly. His once white pants are now splotched with his own color of red. A bundle of gauze has been taped under the right jaw on his neck. I pull it off and see a 10 cm laceration running neatly from right under the angle of his jaw to behind his ear. It's about 5 cm deep and oozing a lot! I push the compresses back in the gaping wound and the bleeding stops. It doesn't appear to have touched any major vessels. He's breathing normally.

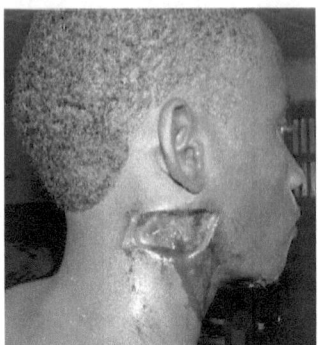

Knife wound to neck

"Nathaniel, come and push on this as hard as you can...right there in the center of the wound...that's it. Don't let go!"

Nurses and volunteers are putting up IV fluids everywhere and frantically mixing up antibiotics.

"Jacob, you and Jason...oh, *et Abel, toi aussi*...go get the gurney from surgery...*ABEL...LE BRANCARD...AU BLOC!*" I keep forgetting Abel is almost deaf. He's one of our hardest workers, though, and was recently made chief of the OR.

"Jacob, never mind, Jason and Abel can get the gurney. Here, take my keys and bring me the ultrasound from my office."

I briefly look at two other women who are beat up. They have a lot of bruises, but are not critical. One is pregnant. Jacob has brought the ultrasound so I check and confirm that the fetus is doing well.

Ansley walks in with a baby strapped to her back. "Her mom's been killed," she reports. "She's not injured at all luckily. We just thought so at first because she was covered with blood."

"*C'est bon!*" I reply as I move off on crutches to the operating room.

In the theater, there's no power. I hobble into the back room and flip on the back-up battery power.

Nurses and volunteers scramble around. IVs are up and flowing in. Needles, syringes, gauze, scalpels, instruments, suture, gloves, scissors, razors, shaved braids, and blood, blood, blood lie scattered everywhere.

Abel takes a razor blade and shaves the hair off the head of the critically injured pregnant woman. The hair has probably taken a lifetime to grow that long. Samedi starts suturing up the huge upside down V-shaped gash in her scalp. She starts to moan as she regains consciousness.

"Siméon," I call out. "Get some Ketamine and Diazepam and put her under."

Aimée now quietly reminds me of a baby with anemia that no one has been able to find an IV on all day. I'd tried an intra-osseous line earlier with a regular 18G needle. We have no specific IO needles. The needles kept bending and I was unsuccessful. I gave up and sent the baby back to the hospital where the nurses continued to search for IV access. A few minutes later, the wounded started pouring in and I forgot about the baby. Now, the baby is in front of me again.

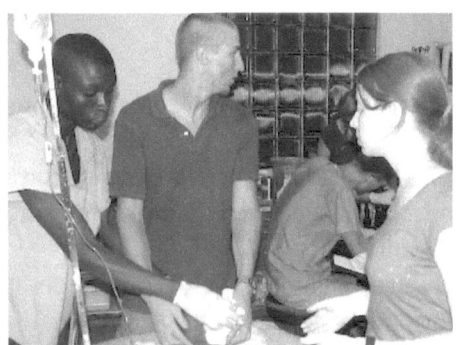

Abel, Jason, James & Kristin

"Jacob, give the baby a milliliter of Ketamine IM and strap him into the Papoose."

The Papoose is a board with padding and straps just the right size to pin a baby down and keep it from moving. Samedi continues suturing. I slice into the baby's ankle and dissect down to the saphenous vein. I find it and slide in an IV catheter. Aimée hooks up the blood. I suture the wound closed.

Now it's time for the young man with the neck wound.

"Kristin, you and Ansley take this baby off to the Pediatric ward. Siméon, you and Jason move the man onto this gurney."

"*Illa Allah bas, kan Allah mafi ana amutu khalas.*" The young man speaks earnestly, recognizing that without God he'd be dead.

"*Al hamdullilah!*" I reply and he nods and closes his eyes as he starts softly repeating verses from the Qur'an.

I stay seated on my stool as Siméon puts him under with Ketamine. Jason washes out the wound. I bring together the subcutaneous tissues with a couple interrupted sutures and close the skin loosely. I'm done.

"ABEL...PANSEMENT!" I point to the gauze bucket and to the man's neck. Abel and I communicate best in our own version of sign language. He nods and takes over.

Emily brings the ultrasound machine into the operating room. I place the probe over the uterus of the woman whose scalp Samedi just stitched up. The fetus has a strong heart beat. Measuring the femur length and bi-parietal diameter reveals a 32 week pregnancy. At 32 weeks the baby will be premature but should be able to survive a quick C-section if the mom dies.

I grab my crutches and swing outside. Sarah is coming from the operating room.

"They've just brought in another guy, a Nangjéré man. The sous-prefect's truck is out looking for other victims. This one doesn't look too bad."

He has some cuts on his hand and a stab wound over his shoulder blade that isn't deep. I leave it for Samedi to suture. I limp home accompanied by the volunteers.

To wind down, we play a game of Settlers of Catan. Just as we start the second game, Ansley knocks at the door.

"More victims have arrived..."

As I approach the hospital, I see bodies scattered all over. Camouflaged gendarmes armed with AK47s are unloading people from a Land Cruiser pick-up. I head straight to the operating room and open the door.

"Bring the worst ones straight in here," I yell over my shoulder. Samedi is just finishing up suturing the last man from the previous wave of wounded.

"James, I just heard an interesting story," begins Samedi. "The guy I just sewed up? He started it all. Here's what happened:

"This Nangjéré man was out in his field and saw some cows eating his rice. He challenged the nomadic herdsman. The herder started to pull out his bow and arrow, so the Nangjéré man rushed him. They grappled for a moment. The nomad pulled out his knife and the farmer grabbed the blade with his hand. He quickly let go and the cattle herdsman stabbed him in the back. The farmer fainted and the other fled.

"The women watching assumed the Nangjéré man was dead," Samedi continues. "So, they ran to the market screaming bloody murder. When their relatives heard that their 'brother' was dead, they attacked a group of nomad women just leaving the market.

"Now both sides were on the prowl. A group of Nangjéré headed to the nomad village going from door to door dragging women and children out and beating them up. The cattlemen are now organizing reprisals. There aren't enough gendarmes to control the numbers of fighters, so they are just picking up bodies."

Samedi finishes and wheels the man outside where he quietly slips into the night.

Now Abel brings in a wiry man who looks like Kobe Bryant. He has a huge slash across his right lower chest. It's about 25cm long and goes all the way down to the ribs that God gave him to protect his liver and lungs.

Another victim is a leathery, middle-aged man with cuts all over. His main complaint is they've taken out his left eye. I ask him to remove the rags covering his face. I now see a 10cm slash across his cheek leaving his left eye swollen shut. Small lacerations cover his body and arms.

Another man shows me his finger. There is an open dislocation. I quickly pop it back in joint. He also has a stab wound to his leg which has cracked his tibia.

I reduce the tibia fracture, flush out the wound with diluted bleach, slosh some Betadine on a piece of gauze and place it over the gash.

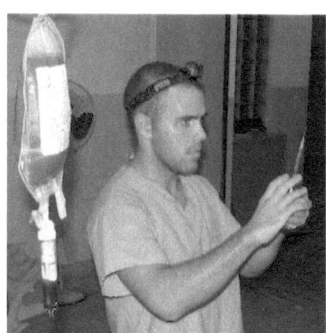
Jacob

"Jacob, hold that tight," I order. "Jason, keep pulling on his leg so we don't lose the reduction. *Abel...Abel? AAAAHHHBBBELLLLL! Platre... PLATRE...PLAAAAAAATTTRRRE!!!*" He doesn't understand even when I gesture. Finally, I point him to the wound and he holds pressure on it.

"Jacob, go get all the casting materials. Just like we did last Saturday night: web roll, tubing, plaster, a basin of water, scissors," I then turn to Siméon and point to the man with the chest wound. "Siméon, Diazepam and Ketamine for this guy too."

"Ashadu anna la ilah illa Allah, wa ashadu anna Muhammadan rasul Ullah." The man repeats the Muslim creed over and over until he starts to drift off. Then he tenses up, holding his breath: a Ketamine reaction.

"Sarah, get me some Chlorpromazine." She can't find it.

"Someone get me some from the Pharmacy."

"There is none," replies Samedi. "I needed some last night and couldn't find it. We're all out."

Just then Sarah comes out of the main operating room, "I found one ampoule."

The man finally relaxes and starts breathing. His oxygen saturation climbs back slowly to normal. I do a running subcutaneous suture to bring the muscles and fascia back together. I close the skin loosely with interrupted sutures. I want the wound to drain since it's contaminated.

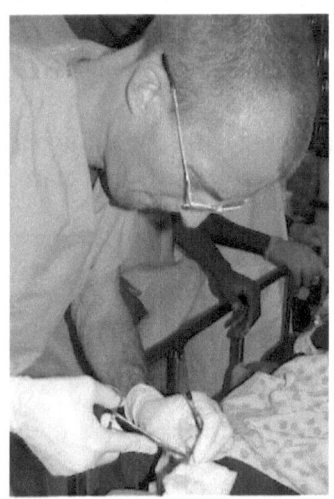

James the Cripple

"ABEL...PANSEMENT!" I point to the wound and then to the box of gauze sponges. Abel nods and smiles. Jacob has arrived with the casting materials. I want to finish the cast while Samedi finishes suturing up all the other lacerations.

Kristin, Ansley and Augustin are working on another man just brought in by the gendarmes on a stretcher.

"His intestine is sticking out his side and he's got a ton of cuts," reports Kristin.

"Ok, Kristin, start an IV with Ringers. Siméon, Ampicillin 2g, Gentamicin four ampoules, Flagyl two bottles! Augustin, urinary catheter. Abel, nasogastric tube!"

I turn back to the man with the broken leg. Jacob has already wrapped it well in cotton. I wet the plaster and quickly wind it around the leg while Jason holds it in position.

"Hold it there until it's dry."

I turn to the guy on the stretcher, now parked on the floor. IV fluids are running and antibiotics are in.

"Siméon, start the generator. Let's move him into the main operating room."

I scrub my hands and arms and a few minutes later hop into the OR on one foot. I dry off my hands with an OR towel. Abel helps me with my gown and gloves. The room is lit by just the two overhead operating room lights focused on the prepped abdomen. Jacob slips me my stool. I rest my right knee on it and stand by the right side of the patient. Abel and I spread out the surgical drape. Augustin prays.

I open up his abdomen from his sternum to his belly button and dark blood surges out. Abel suctions it up and I start exploring. There's no major bleeder anywhere. In fact, I don't see any injury. The liver is fine. There is no stool in the abdomen. The stomach and intestines are undamaged.

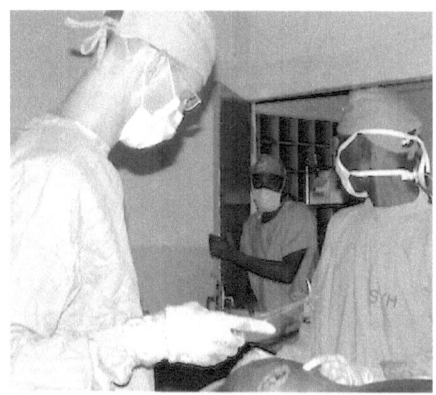

James, Siméon & Abel

I pull out the omentum which is what had come out his side and cut off the contaminated part, tying off the vessels. I can now examine the spleen. I'm surprised to see no damage to that either. Where's the blood coming from?

I get Abel to retract a little deeper. I finally get a good look at the wound. I see air and blood spurting into the abdomen with each breath. *Of course!* I realize. *The bleeding is coming from his lung through a punctured diaphragm!*

I suture up the diaphragmatic tear. Abel suctions out as much blood as possible. I recheck the spleen and it's undamaged. The stab wound left a 3cm laceration in the diaphragm right over the spleen without touching it. I leave a drain in the abdomen and close up.

Then, I insert a chest tube, hear the welcome rush of released air and hook him up to water-seal so his lung can inflate. I suture up the large gash on his arm and the three small gashes on his back.

Jacob and Abel hold the patient as we roll him on his right side. The wound on his buttock is 15cm long, 10cm deep and very bloody. I use a huge needle to bring the deep muscles together and sew the fascia shut. I loosely approximate the skin with interrupted stitches. Abel and Siméon dress all the wounds.

I get home a half hour after midnight. At 1:00am I hear the gendarmes' pick up drive up again. I wait anxiously for a few minutes but no one comes knocking on my door. I fall back asleep. At 6:00am my haggard, yet still beautiful, wife shakes me awake.

"Well, they brought in a bunch more Arab women but they all only have minor injuries so I didn't wake you. They also brought in three more bodies. Do you want to continue antibiotics or anything else on that guy you operated on?"

Oh yeah, post-op orders would be nice, I think. Sarah smilingly holds out an operating room order sheet that I quickly fill out.

She comes back home at 8:00am and shows me a lab slip with her name on it. "Yeah, not only was that the craziest night shift I've ever done, but I had malaria the whole time!"

An hour later, I limp over to the hospital on my crutches to see the patients. Everyone is doing well. All the women are awake. Despite the pain and swelling, all are able to sit up and take some water. Both the man with neck laceration and and the man with the chest wound are also awake and praising Allah. The man with the punctured lung is stable but not awake yet.

Suddenly, a large group of robed and turbaned Arabs fbws in accompanied by soldiers with machine guns. They go through the courtyard and out the back gate to the morgue. I continue to the ER to see the other patients who arrived after I'd gone back to bed.

I've just started rounds when Djibrine, the nurse in charge of supervising our district's health centers comes in.

"The governor and the sous-prefect want to see all the wounded."

I find them in the wards surrounded by Arabs and gendarmes. The sous-prefect sends most of the crowd out leaving a couple guards for the governor. I give them a tour. They write down everyone's name, catalogue their injuries and put them either on the Nangjéré or Arab list.

I finally make it home at noon and my ankle has ballooned to twice it's normal size.

01 November 2008
Lifeless

I squat on the ground outside the operating room. A thin Muslim man squats in front of me, his green Arabic robe pulled tightly across his knees as he hugs them with his arms. He is staring at the blue basin between us. The inside of the basin is covered with a blood-soaked, brightly-patterned yellow wrap around skirt. I lift up the cloth with a gloved hand covered with dried blood. Underneath is a dead infant with a huge, hydrocephalic head. His blank eyes stare up at us as his neck bends back at an impossible angle. Underneath is the placenta still attached to the child by the umbilical cord. All is cold, lifeless and bloody.

I do my best to explain to him in Arabic what happened. "The child, dead, when arrived, dead already. The head, big, not come out. The house of the child broken, the child come out here," I point to my stomach. "Blood come out, a lot, here also. The woman there, she not have much blood when she arrive, not have. See there is not much blood, she found death."

"Both of them, the two of them, both dead?" The man asks in disbelief.

"Yes, both dead, all dead," I repeat as a hundred images from the last two hours flash through my mind...

"Docteur, docteur!"

I slowly stumble out of a deep sleep filled with pleasant dreams. "Yeah, what is it?" I mumble.

"C'est moi, Aimée, I have a case to present to you."

"Ok, I'm coming." I pull on a pair of scrub bottoms and feel my way through the dark to the door and out onto the porch. Aimée is standing outside the screen door with a headlamp on her forehead and a *carnet* along with some other papers in her hand.

"There's a woman, referred, in labor for two days..." Aimée stumbles through presenting the woman. She is one of our laziest nurses and often does as little as possible. I'm a little irritated.

"Whoa, whoa! Start over...no never mind, just give me that!" I take the labor and delivery sheet. I glance quickly over it and it's incomplete. I see the vital signs, heart rate 60/minute, blood pressure 100/70, temperature 37 degrees Celsius. I'll regret later not noticing how generically normal they were.

"*Eh? C'est quoi?*" A voice comes from the room next to us where Jacques has been sleeping. Dr. Jacques has just arrived from Togo freshly graduated from medical school.

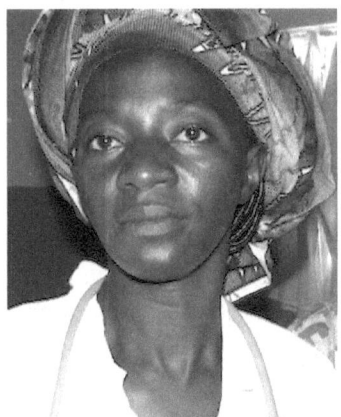

Aimée

"I'm talking to Dr. James," replies Aimée. Jacques quickly appears outside just as I'm giving Aimée some instructions.

"Go back and get more information. Then, come back to see me with the chart completely filled out."

Jacques joins Aimée and they walk off together. I almost yell after them to tell them to check a hemoglobin. I catch myself, thinking *I'll be over to see her shortly anyway.* This is the second thing I later regret not doing.

I go back to my room and decide to lie down. It's been a long week. I've done a lot of surgeries. I also started training village health care workers to give HIV and tuberculosis medicines under directly observed therapy. I'll just close my eyes for a few minutes until Aimée and Jacques get back. *Voila!* The third thing I later regret.

"*Docteur? Docteur?*" The gentle voice of Jacques floats across my subconscious. I go to the door. I glance up at the clock. It reads 4:25am. I didn't look at the clock when Aimée first came. But, I did hear the fridge running which it's scheduled to do four hours a day starting at 6:00am, noon, 6:00pm and midnight. So, three to four hours have passed since I saw Aimée and Jacques walking off together. A strange sense of foreboding falls over me.

"I've examined the woman and I think she has a ruptured uterus," says Jacques.

"Go call Abel and Dr. Franklin," I urge. "I'll be right there."

I pull on a scrub top, grab my keys and fly out the door. I stop by the other house real quick to make sure Franklin's awake. Once he's awake, I make my way across the compound to the labor and delivery room.

I walk in the room. I see Abré in a white coat standing by the bed. When I glance at the patient, my heart skips a beat. A tiny Arabic woman lies stretched out on the table with one knee bent in the air. Blood has pooled between her legs. An IV with Glucose and Oxytocin is dripping into her left arm. Her thin abdomen is grossly distorted with several large, abnormal looking lumps. But what arrests my attention is when I look at her face.

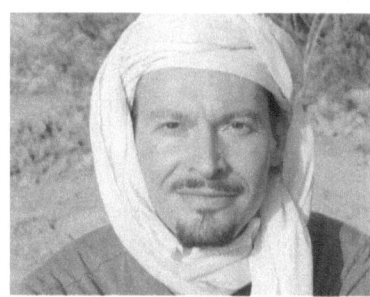

Franklin

Her head flops to one side and her eyes are rolled back in her head. She is pale and her only breaths are occasional sighs. She is on death's door and I see it instantly. I quickly feel for her heartbeat which is present but slow. I flip down her eyelids with my finger and my blood freezes. Her conjunctiva are white. She has practically bled to death in our hospital.

"Aimée, quick call the lab, we need blood! Abré, run and get me some Ringers!"

Franklin arrives and quickly starts looking for a better IV. She stops breathing. I start chest compressions. Franklin has found an IV in her neck. We get fluids running. Abel arrives. We take turns with CPR.

"Franklin, what about the monitor from the operating room?" He runs and quickly brings back the monitor: no blood pressure and a weak O2 sat.

Finally, after what seems like hours the lab guy arrives.

"Abré, what blood type are you?"

"O positive."

"Mathieu, just check to see if she's positive or negative and if she's positive Abré will give."

She is B positive. Jacques and Abré run off to donate a bag of blood each. Aimée is B positive and refuses to give. Abel and I keep up the chest compressions while Franklin maintains her airway. We get the first bag which is only a third full of Abré's blood. Franklin hangs it up.

"Abel, you and Abré get the stretcher and lets take her to the operating room."

We flop her bloodied body onto the stretcher. Abel and Abré carry her quickly to the operating room. I continue chest compressions. Franklin carries the blood and IV's.

We get her all set up on the operating room table with blood splashed everywhere. The patient is still pulseless so we continue our resuscitation. I hope that if we can keep her oxygen circulating until we replace her blood loss, maybe we can still save her.

We try some Atropine to start her heart. We try shocking her. Nothing. We have no Adrenaline. Then I remember we have some spinal kits. I open up two kits so we can use the adrenaline inside. Nothing works, but we continue CPR.

Finally, a third bag of blood is running. I decide to take out the baby. Abel sloshes Betadine on the belly. I quickly open up a C-section kit. Abel and I put on gowns and sterile gloves. One slash and I'm in the belly. I cut the baby's face, but he's dead already. His head is five times normal size: hydrocephalus. That's why he couldn't come out.

Her uterus is in tatters. I pull out the baby and placenta. I clamp across what's left of the uterus and cut it out. I tie off the clamps, dump some Celox in the pelvis and hold pressure for five minutes. The whole thing takes about 15 minutes. All the donated blood has run in. We've been working on her for almost two hours. She still is flatlined.

"Stop CPR," I say wearily and go out to tell her husband.

I'm kneeling in front of the Muslim husband. I just told him his wife and the unborn child between us are dead. I'm not sure how he'll react. A brief image flashes through my mind of the violence of two weeks ago: Arabs stabbing and killing Africans and vice versa. I recall the chaos in the hospital as we tried to save as many as possible.

But there is no revenge taken on me today. Instead, a gentle chanting in classic Arabic rises from the depths of his sorrowed heart.

"*La ilah illa Allah. La ilah illa Allah.*" He repeats the Muslim creed over and over. It seems to soothe his sorrow. "*Al hamdullilah!*" A Muslim brother from Lai comes and kneels down beside. They recite some surahs from the Qur'an in a low voice.

"Find me some Muslim brothers here," says the bereaved man. "All the believers here in the hospital." The other Muslim goes off. Soon a small group of robed and turbaned men surrounds us.

"Would you like to see your wife?" I ask.

He nods and we go into the operating room. Abel and Jacques have been cleaning. A portly Arab with a beige robe and white turban accompanies us. The woman is lying on the stretcher covered with a black Muslim dress. Intricate Arabic designs in gold are woven into the fabric. The husband uncovers the wife's face and asks for water.

"*Almi...almi.*"

I get some water from the faucet and bring it to him in a small basin.

"Put a little over my hands," he asks me in Arabic.

I pour water over his right hand. He uses it to gently wash and wipe down his dead wife's face closing her eyes. The other Arab also moves his hand down the face to close the eyes. Then they cover her back up. As we take her out to the morgue, I hear some low sobs coming from back in the operating room.

Fifteen minutes later, the brothers from the Mosque arrive. I carefully explain in broken Arabic what happened.

"*Xalas!*"

"*Mashallah!*"

"*Al hamdullilah!*"

The men comfort and console the husband. They take the body off to be appropriately buried as soon as possible. She will be placed on her right side facing Mecca as tradition demands.

I go home.

02 November 2008

Mistake

I'm sure the elderly man has a gallbladder problem. I'm no ultrasound expert, but there is obviously something inside that gall bladder that shouldn't be there. Besides, he complains of pain right over that spot that is worse when he eats. Plus, his bilirubin is elevated, another sign that could point to a gall bladder problem.

I'm hesitant to operate. He's a friend. In fact, he is the local chief here in Béré. His name is Totho Timothée. His brother is a motorcycle taxi-man. He takes us back and forth to Kélo when our car isn't running or the roads are impassible due to the rains.

In the end, I decide surgery is the right thing to do. I'm sure he needs an operation for his gallbladder. I'm wrong.

I stand to his right side. Franklin has given him a high spinal anesthetic. I plan on making a somewhat relaxed incision just below his ribs on the right. We pray. I start cutting. Abel and Jacques assist. Since it's a big case, I have set up the electrocautery. Soon the smell of barbecuing human flesh fills the room as I burn through the abdominal muscles before entering the peritoneal cavity.

It's 110 degrees outside. The A/C is on. Jacques, however, is not used to Tchadian heat. Togo is relatively cooler. Sweat runs in rivulets down Jacques face. I usually don't notice my own sweat until after surgery when I pull off my gown and notice that my scrubs are soaked.

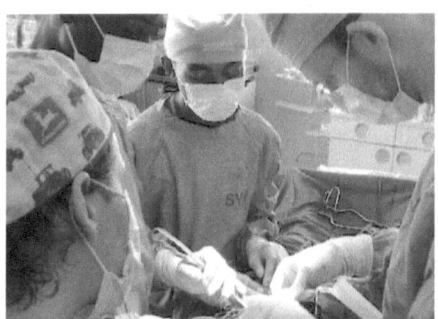
Franklin, Abel, Jacques & James

I have Abel retract the liver gently. I get a good look at the gallbladder. It looks normal. I pinch it between my fingers. It feels normal. I'm starting to feel sheepish. There is ascites. I look closer at the liver. He has advanced liver cirrhosis.

Of course the bilirubin was elevated! I shouldn't have operated! I might have even endangered his life. Better close and get out of here before I do more harm.

Then I notice something out of the corner of my eye that gives me pause.

"Jacques, pull the stomach back a little again. Yeah, just like that."

I see a small black spot on the first part of the duodenum. Before my brain can even run through a differential diagnosis, the spot starts to open. A stream of clear, gooey liquid wells up out of the wound. A duodenal ulcer just perforated before my very eyes!

Abel quickly aspirates up the stomach acid with the suction tip. I call for some suture. I place several interrupted sutures along the edge of the ulcer. I leave them untied till I have a whole row ready to close. I pull some of the omentum back from the stomach edge and lay it across the perforation. I tie the sutures across the omentum patching up the hole. I irrigate profusely while Jacques suctions continuously. I then close up the muscle, fascia and skin of the abdominal wall.

I just made a mistake that saved my friend's life. If I hadn't mistakenly misread the ultrasound, I wouldn't have operated. If I hadn't mistakenly thought it was the gallbladder, I wouldn't have made the perfect incision to allow me to see and close the ulcer. If I'd have waited half and hour more, it would have perforated letting stomach acid pour into the abdomen leading to all kinds of complications. If it had happened a day or two before I did the operation, he'd probably be dead already.

24 November 2008
Progress

I'm back in Moundou to check on the progress of the remodeling of the old mission house. A month ago we finally got the squatters out and Antoine introduced me to Frederic, a self-made builder who did some work on the Moundou Adventist Junior High School. I saw some of Frederic's other work and was impressed. Antoine assured me he is humble and honest.

As soon as the money from the Loma Linda Women's Auxiliary came in to the bank, I gave Frederic a generous sum to start the remodeling. He knocked out the bricks blocking the old windows, removed the wall between the back two rooms, tore off the roof and ceiling, extended the roof over a new back veranda, and poured a new slab for the deck.

Looking at the house, I'm already encouraged. Just having the old ceiling and roof off makes it seem cleaner and bigger. Sunlight pours in through the enlarged windows into the new huge back room through the leaves of the mango and guava trees surrounding the house.

The next phase will be to wall off the property to give us some privacy and increased security. There is a lot more criminal activity in a city like Moundou compared to a village like Béré.

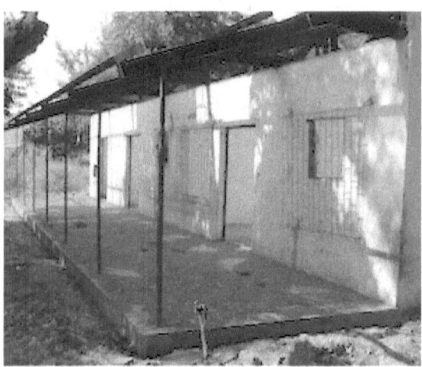

Moundou Surgery Center project

I hear the call to prayer over a loud speaker from a local mosque. The project is in a Muslim neighborhood in this mostly Christian southern town. Down the street is one of two bakeries in town. The local Soccer field is right in front. Directly across the road is a military base with a brewery to the right and a cigarette factory to the left.

I can't think of a more perfect place for a Surgery Center!

27 November 2008

Thanksgiving

When I came to Moundou a few days ago, I'd stopped at the post office in Kélo. I'd found 14 packages waiting for our volunteers so I paid for them, loaded them in the van and continued to Moundou.

Now, I'm on my way back to Béré. Frédéric, our builder, rides with us back so he can look over the operating room in Béré to better understand what we're looking for. Back on the dirt road to Béré, I have a wonderful idea. Little do I know how much deception I will have to employ in order for it to succeed.

The first thing is to swear our driver, Levi, to secrecy. Then we have to quickly unload the packages into my house without the volunteers seeing them. I'm not going to tell them I've picked up their packages until

Thanksgiving morning. Our volunteers are desperate to have those goodies.

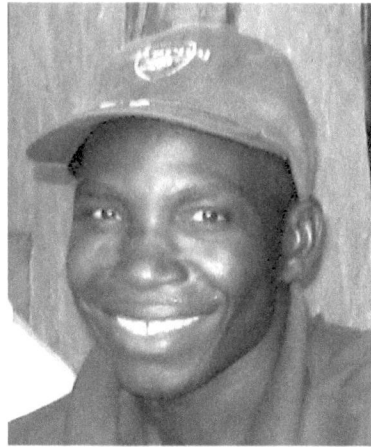

Levi

The very next day, Stefan comes to see me. "I've arranged everything with André. He's given me the day off so I can go to Kélo to see if we have any packages. Some of our families have sent us things to make Thanksgiving dinner with."

I put on my most severe boss face. "Stefan, did you come here to work, or to get packages. You should've told me yesterday. I passed right by the post-office and could've easily checked to see if there was anything for you guys. We're really busy right now. Besides, how are you going to get a bunch of packages back on a *moto*? It's just not a good idea. I'll probably be making another trip early next week, I can pick them up then."

Stefan's face falls, but he has no choice but to accept.

"Well, ok, but Kristin was going to go with me, maybe she can just go. She's not scheduled till this evening so she wouldn't miss work."

Thinking quickly, I'm a little frightened at how easily I continue the deception. "Stefan, do you really think it's a good idea for a girl to go by herself to Kélo? It's just not very smart. It'll be even harder for her to carry all those packages back. Plus, this is Tchad, it could be dangerous." I'm lying through my teeth, but somehow keep a straight, concerned face.

Stefan turns sadly away to go back to his accounting office. I smile inwardly at my success. It is short lived as lies tend to pile on top of each other. Once you start it's hard to stop.

I have to tell a bunch more to Kristin later on. She is unwilling to accept Stefan's explanation. She feels that if she talks to me personally, maybe this mean boss will change his mind. I hold firm and try to convince her it's just not a good idea.

"Besides, there's other things already planned. It won't be a real Thanksgiving anyway. We might as well just wait and have our Thanksgiving next week sometime."

She's crestfallen, but there's nothing she can do.

Tuesday night, I'm chatting with Kristin and Ansley. Unfortunately, they've come up with a solution that I can't lie my way out of. I'm forced to spill the beans. They are excited, but agree with me to keep it a secret from the others. Ansley joins in the lying on Wednesday when everyone else is together.

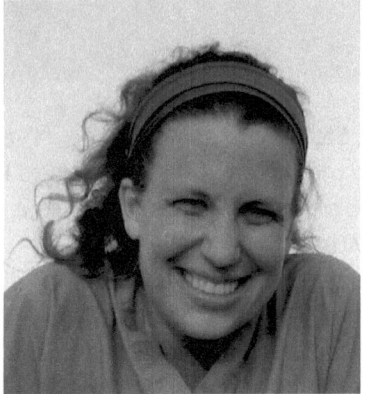

Ansley

"I had explosive diarrhea six times last night. I'm just not up to a trip to Kélo...and Emily shouldn't go by herself," she announces.

Early Thursday morning, I pull the 14 packages and numerous letters out of my closet and carry them over to the volunteers' common room in the middle house. I leave a note that says, "Ho! Ho! Ho! Merry Thanksgiving! Merry Thanksgiving!" However, it almost doesn't turn out very merry at all.

I start work on Thanksgiving morning with rounds on a completely full hospital. There are no empty beds. Then, I do a tubal ligation, a D & C plus tubal ligation on another woman, excision of a rectal polyp on an eight year old Arab boy, a bilateral inguinal hernia repair with mosquito net on an elderly man and another emergency D & C for an incomplete spontaneous abortion. Finally, I finish at 4:30pm just in time to go to the going away party for Salomon, one of our nurses.

I slip into the courtyard where Salomon's friends and many of the staff are already seated on a variety of chairs, stools and mats. I slip off my Crocs and settle onto a mat. My ankle is aching a little and somewhat swollen after a long day upright in the operating room, but it's not too bad. I exchange pleasantries with Job and Koumakoy. I nod at Siméon and Abel who've spent all day in surgery with me.

Salomon slides onto the mat next to me and we have some decent small talk as Jason serves us the best *bouillie* I've had in Tchad. Jason contracted with our cook, Zachée, for the feast. This *bouillie* is a rice porridge with milk, sugar, cinnamon and peanut paste. I grab the crude metal bowl from Jason and slurp it up without a spoon.

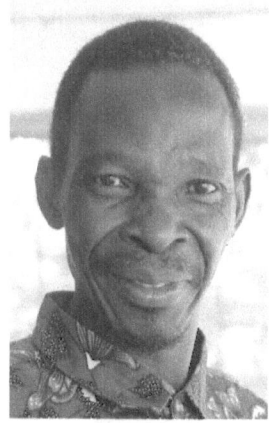

Zachée

The second course is roasted chicken in a tomato sauce with boiled sweet potatoes, all served over mushy rice. It's quite tasty, but I'm trying to save room for Thanksgiving dinner later on.

At 6:00pm, we all head to my house to prepare the feast. We have invited Gary and Wendy and their volunteers—Steve, Jeremy and Annie. Gary and Wendy just got back with their kids, Kaleb and Cherise, after being gone for six months. We also have six student volunteers, a Danish high school student named Maria, Sarah and I. Sarah, however, has volunteered for the night shift. Being Danish, American Thanksgiving doesn't mean much to her at all.

Jacob's mom has sent five packages stuffed with everything we need for a feast. The menu is impressive: Fri-Chik, powdered garlic mashed potatoes, gravy, cranberry sauce, relish, pasta salad, stuffing, spiced apple cider, candied yams, and a pumpkin pie spiced squash dessert with real whipped cream! Gary and Wendy add some real mashed potatoes, more gravy, a cranberry-like hibiscus flower sauce, and some stuffing made from scratch. Jeremy and Annie bring fresh squeezed lemonade, boiled beets and a fresh garden salad of tomatoes, lettuce, cucumbers and sprouts.

Jacob's mom has also sent Thanksgiving-themed plates, napkins and decorations. With the pumpkin-like squash in the center of the table we're only missing NFL football to make it feel like a real American holiday.

Right before eating, Sarah comes over to tell me that she's already hospitalized five kids with malaria, three of them with severe anemia needing blood transfusions. Luckily, Samedi is on with her until 9:00pm so they've got everything under control. However, the hospital is now full again despite being cleared out by me in the morning. Sarah refuses my offer to eat with us, saying she'd rather I just brought her something later. She goes back to work.

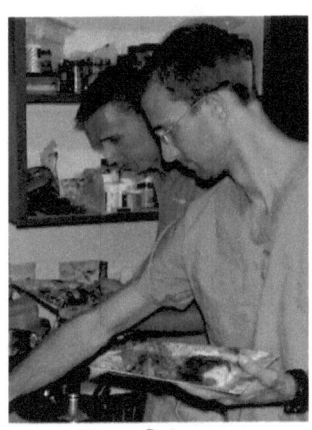

Gary & James

We all sit down around the table. Before eating, we go around and each person says five things they're thankful for; one for each of the five kernels of corn placed before them. We pray and then chow down.

Just as I'm finishing my overloaded plate Hortence, the midwife, comes knocking.

"There's a woman, eight months pregnant with vaginal bleeding," she says. "She was referred from the health center two days ago, but just came now."

I wipe my mouth, change into scrubs and go to labor and delivery. The woman is severely anemic. Hortence already had Mathieu check a hemoglobin and it comes back 4.8 g/dl. She has a placenta previa where the placenta wants to come out before the baby. I think I find a fetal heart beat.

We quickly start two large bore IV's, start rapid fluid resuscitation, give her antibiotics, and take her to the operating room. Fortunately, her blood type is AB+ making her a universal recipient. Mathieu takes blood from both her brother and father while we prep her for surgery.

Siméon does the anesthesia. He starts the first bag of blood running as I pull out a dead baby. The boy's skin is already peeling off meaning he died a few days ago. Fortunately, there's not much bleeding. We quickly close up as the second transfusion runs in. Her heartbeat is almost normal now and her blood pressure has come up. We wheel her into the wards almost running over some Arab women who've spread their sleeping mats right across the entrance. We are forced to leave her on the gurney for the night since there are no available beds.

I come home at about 10:00pm. I join in the games of Settlers of Catan and Citadels. We play until almost two in the morning when I fall into a deep, contented sleep.

A Happy Thanksgiving indeed!

30 November 2008
Morning

It's early morning and I can't sleep again. This time, though, it's because I'm excited. For the first time in several weeks, I'll actually be doing something. My ankle wound has turned into a non-healing tropical ulcer. It has kept me from doing anything except the bare minimum.

Every morning, I go up to the hospital, quickly see the hospitalized patients, do all the scheduled surgeries and then retire home to elevate my swollen foot. My day revolves around how fast I can get home to make the swelling go down, do a dressing change and take antibiotics. I even got so scared for a few days that I had Sarah start an IV on me and give me antibiotic injections.

This morning, though, my ankle seems to have turned the corner. Today, I'm going flying with Gary to N'Djamena. I've needed to go to N'Djamena for a while, but with my wound the idea of a eight hour, bumpy ride in the back of a Toyota mini-bus isn't that appealing. In

Gary's plane, getting to N'Djamena has turned into a two hour pleasant flight over the African plain.

It's still dark, but I can't sleep anyway. I get up and fix breakfast. I fry up some day old rice and beans with little bit of curry. Not a typical American breakfast, but sometimes you have to eat for strength and not for sport.

The roosters have been crowing since 3:00am, the dogs have been barking and the drums have just stopped. The morning seems more quiet and peaceful than normal. Just the lulling, rhythmic sound of crickets break the early dawn's silence. I step outside into the desert cold. I quickly go back in and put on a sweatshirt. I pull my small North Face backpack over the sweatshirt and slip on my Crocs.

My ankle is a little stiff, but it feels good to be out on the deep, sandy road towards Béré's laterite airstrip. It's a two kilometer walk. I have the village mostly to myself at this hour.

An early morning mist rests over the tops of the thatch-roofed, brownish-red clay huts. The only ones awake are a few women pounding millet in homemade wooden mortars with six feet long wooden pestles. The *dooomp, dooomp* of the pounding of grain into the base for the typical Tchadian breakfast porridge echos across the stillness.

A few children are also up trying to chase away the night's chill around hastily gathered grass and stick fires. Their dark faces hidden behind the white smoke wafting from the incompletely dried weed fires break into toothy grins as they see *Nasara* walking gingerly away from the hospital.

They are mostly dressed in ragged shorts, holey pants and torn t-shirts. It's no wonder they're cold. The dry season has descended upon us leaving us with up to 40 degrees Fahrenheit difference between day and night temperatures. The luscious greenness of the rainy season has rapidly evaporated into the brown, dead, dusty dryness of the majority of the year here in the heart of Africa.

I approach some of them, who eye me warily with looks of mixed curiosity and fear. I extend my hand, palm up. Several of the bigger, braver ones approach to shake hands. I shake my head and show them how to give me "five".

"*Tag kebeng,*" I encourage them in Nangjéré. When they finally get up the courage to try, everyone wants to get in on the action. They all start giggling and laughing. What fun to really smack hard the palm of a grown-up, even more so when it's *Nasara's*!

I finally get to the airstrip where the early morning sunrise colors the mostly white plane with a tinge of pink. Gary tests the oil and fuel levels then fills up the wing tanks with his bright red cans of Cameroonian gasoline. A few kids have gathered around, but not as many as usual since it's still so early. Gary sits down with his family to eat breakfast.

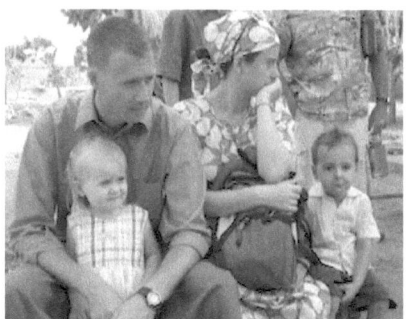
Gary, Cherise, Wendy & Kaleb

After breakfast, Gary says good-bye to Wendi, Kaleb & Cherise and we head back out to the airstrip.

Soon we slide into the tiny Cessna loaded up with empty fuel and propane containers. After a short taxi we are soaring up and over Béré where the 10,000 inhabitants of this Tchadian county seat disappear quickly into the groves of mango trees. The occasional glimpses of thatch or tin-roofed houses give us a clue that there's actually a village hidden in this vast plain. We bank over the hospital to get a good aerial view. It also seems so small and insignificant when seen from on high.

N'Djamena, here we come.

07 December 2008

Ma Joie

I hardly get any sleep. I wake up at 3:00am before falling back asleep until the alarm sounds at 4:30am.

"Sarah, I think I'm not going to N'Djamena. What am I really going to do there anyway? I'll just stay here."

Sarah rises and gets ready while I lie in bed. At 4:55am, Levi still hasn't arrived. I get up and drive our 4x4 Toyota Hiace minibus over to the hospital. I flip on the lights in the men's ward.

"*As-salaamu aleikum!* Wake up! We're leaving at five, remember? You're supposed to be ready!"

Our two friends, Mahamat and Lamglé, slowly get up, wiping the sleep from their eyes. Their *gardes-malades* start pulling down the mosquito nets and taking off the sheets carefully from underneath the two men. Both of their right legs are casted from groin to ankle.

Last week, I performed the second surgery on each of them for non-healing femur fractures. They are relatives and both were in motorcycle accidents. I tried doing an open reduction and traction for each of them, but it didn't work. I just operated again and put in plates and screws with a cast. Now, I want to take them to N'Djamena for x-rays since our machine hasn't been working for years. Besides, they live there and this way they can convalesce at home.

I'm now awake. Since Levi still isn't here I decide last minute to go to N'Djamena. I quickly pack, open the fridge and grab some cold Tchadian pizza and a week old bottle of vanilla protein drink for the road. Levi still hasn't arrived so we hit the road without him.

Driving in the dark with headlights actually makes it easier on the rain scourged roads as the shadows light up where the holes are. Dawn breaks and a cool desert morning rushes in the open windows.

I startle a brightly colored bird with several shades of brilliant blue and a super-long tail. Unfortunately, it isn't fast enough and gets taken out in mid flight by the left side of the minibus' grill. He dies with a quick crunch.

Driving in Tchad means constant vigilance to miss the countless sheep, goats, horses, cattle, camels, bicycles and pedestrians sharing the narrow roads. Arab donkey caravan brings me almost to a halt on a one-way bridge. As I come to a complete stop, one of the dumb asses with a piece of wood strapped to it's side turns into the car. With a crinkle of glass my left headlight is no more.

Moving on past the bridge, two little baby goats, one black and one white with black spots streak suddenly across the highway. They are just evenly enough spaced to simultaneously be crunched, one under each front wheel. I glance in the rearview mirror and see the white one motionless. The black one struggles with it's head and front legs while it's back legs lie stuck to the asphalt.

Rounding the corner onto the bridge at the entrance to N'Djamena, we strain to catch a glimpse of the hippos in the river but to no avail. I drive through town and drop off Mahamat and Lamglé at the National Reference Hospital. The ER is chaotic filled with bodies in various stages of being treated with casts, dressings, bandages, IV fluids and shots.

Nasara Encore

Sarah and I bounce around N'Djamena in the Hiace to the National Center for Tuberculosis over near the airport. We are trying to get more meds. The secretary tells us to wait in the Pharmacy.

A lean, lighter-skinned Tchadian with a six-o'clock shadow beard and a bright smile waves us into his office. He orders a young boy to bring *chai* while he fills our medication order.

His French isn't that great. When we speak a few words of Arabic he lights up. He speaks clearly and slowly so we can understand, peppering his talk with the occasional French or English word.

Apparently, he did all his primary and secondary schooling here in Tchad, but in Arabic instead of French. It's possible to go through school here without learning French, but unusual. He then studied three years of nursing and three years of pharmacy in Syria.

"Christians and Muslims are very similar," he continues as we nod in agreement. "We don't drink alcohol or eat pork."

"We don't either," I say in agreement. "And we don't smoke either."

He nods, impressed.

"The most important thing in life is to make it to paradise," I add.

"Inshallah, inshallah," he says hopefully. "We believe in all the holy books: *at-Tawrat, al-Injil, wal-Qur'an.* They all are God's way of communicating with *al-Insan.*"

"The true religion," I add, "is the religion of *Ibrahim.*"

He nods again. Pointing to Sarah and I, he asks, "Are you married?"

"Yes," replies Sarah. "But only to each other. *Adoum* had only *Hawa* and not *Maryam, Khadidja,* etc..."

"In Islam," he says laughing, "it is permitted to have four wives, but only under special circumstances."

"True," I confirm. "In countries hit hard by war, like Tchad, where women outnumber men, I can understand that. But it's an exception and I find I have enough trouble with only one woman, why add more?"

He stretches out his hand to be slapped and grasped in the Tchadian way of sharing a joke as he laughs along with me.

"Yes, that's why I also only have one wife," he concurs. "Besides, life is difficult and who can afford more than one wife anyway? Do you have any children?"

"Not yet," says Sarah.

"Allah will give you many,..." he insists, then adds, "...*inshallah.*"

He then calls the boy back and tells him to pour us some more *chai* as we continue our conversation.

"We have several Qur'ans at home," mentions Sarah.

"*Mashallah,*" he approves. "Are they in English or what?"

"Arabic, English and French," I say. He nods approvingly.

We finish our tea. He helps us haul out the TB meds to the Hiace. We shake hands promising to see each other another day, *inshallah.*

I somehow have no doubt that I will see him again, maybe not on earth, but certainly in paradise.

Sarah and I run some other errands before being called back to pick up Mahamat and Lamglé. We wander through several dirt road detours through the suburbs of N'Djamena until Mahamat tells us to stop. We are in front of a mud plastered, three-room house with a ramshackle, covered dirt porch which Mahamat claims as his. He apologizes saying a huge wind knocked half his wall down last May.

Sarah and I help them out on their crutches and over to a mat in the shade. We are invited to sit with them. A woman places a metal bowl of water before us. I try to ignore the floating things as I bring it slowly to my parched lips. A young boy is sent off for some Cokes and a Grapefruit soda called *Top.* We then have some rice *boule* with some green leaf and dried fish sauce. I'm starving. I dig into the sticky rice paste and dip it into the spicy sauce. I can't eat it fast enough. I don't usually like boule, but for some reason this just hits the spot.

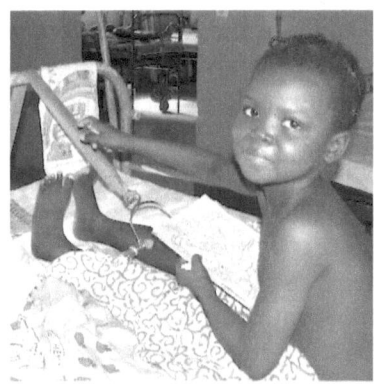

Ma Joie

We head off back downtown and stop at Ma Joie's house. Ma Joie is the eight-year-old girl who also had a non-healing right femur fracture. I also operated on her and put her in traction. The only difference is that she healed after two months and has been home for over a month already. She is also a relative of Mahamat and Lamglé.

We enter a low, dank mud entrance down an open alley past some couches in various stages of fabrication until we turn into an open courtyard. There our shy, cute little friend limps towards us on one crutch. Apparently, she doesn't need it, but her grandfather insisted she use it in front of us in case we expected it.

We greet all 14 members of the extended family. Ma Joie makes my day by lighting up with a crooked tooth grin when I lay out my hand palm up so she can give me "five". She slaps it hard and soon all the other kids are lining up! Right before we leave, she runs off and brings us each a black plastic bag with some brightly colored African cloth as a present.

11 December 2008
Blue baby

Dr. Jacques knocks on my front door.

"I just assisted an uncomplicated vaginal delivery, but the baby is having respiratory distress. The nares are flaring, the intercostal muscles are retracting and he's just having a hard time. I tried aspirating to see if he had any mucus but it seems his nose is blocked. It's like there's just no connection to the throat."

I head over with Jacques. At the hospital I enter a dimly lit corridor. I push open the first door to the right into a brightly lit, but small chamber. A quick glance takes in a young woman lying comfortably on the bed. I don't see much blood around and the new mother is breathing and looking around normally. She's fine.

I turn to the neonatal resuscitation table. I see a chubby, bluish gray baby with a disproportionately tiny head lying staring up and grunting, but not really breathing.

I grab him around the chest, flip him over on my hand and slap him hard on his back. He starts to cry vigorously. I think that must be it. They just are afraid of these supposedly fragile little beings and don't stimulate them enough.

I flp him back over onto the green, brightly patterned cloth underneath him and reach for the aspirator. A tiny tube goes into a small canister with a slightly larger tube coming out the same top. I slip the bigger end in my mouth ready to suck and slide the smaller tube into the baby's nose. It only goes in 1-2 cm and is stuck. I wiggle it around and then try the other nostril. Still no passage.

I stick my finger into the newborn's mouth straight back into his throat. He starts to gag as I feel around and confirm, there's no opening between his nostrils and his airway.

A newborn is an obligatory nose breather. This allows him to nurse and breath at the same time. These are two very important things God makes sure newborns know how to do instinctively, because there's just no spare time to have to learn it. The baby only breaths through his mouth if he cries.

We can't just make him cry all the time, he just won't do it. He cries a little and starts to pink up and then goes back to sucking in impotently on his blocked up nostrils.

What to do? I think quickly and go to the operating room to find some probes and see if there isn't some passage back there after all that's just blocked up. I grab the hemorroidectomy kit as that's the only one I know of with probes. Back in labor and delivery I can't get them to pass. The probes go nowhere.

I call the father in and explain the situation. "He can't breath through his mouth because it's against his instinct and he can't live without breathing. We can try to poke a hole through but he could bleed a lot and die or we could damage some important things, but the bottom line is he won't live if we do nothing. What do you think?"

"Do what you have to, it's in God's hands," he replies.

I grab a Kelly clamp and probe downward in the right nostril to where the palate seems thinnest between the nose and mouth. I poke through. I then do the same on the other side. However, he still can't breath because the mucosa of the mouth just falls back in place. We need something to keep it open.

I grab the aspirator and cut off a piece of the bigger tubing. I reach the clamp through into the mouth, grasp the tube and pull it out through the nose. The first time it pops all the way out. I then attach another clamp onto the mouth and and pull it through again, this time the clamp prevents it from coming all the way out. I repeat it for the other nostril.

I suck up some blood out of the nose and mouth using what's left of the newborn aspirator. He's still struggling but I can hear and feel air coming out the two tubes.

I then insert a feeding tube in the mouth. The mother starts squeezing out breastmilk which we give through the tube with a syringe.

He's already pinking up, only his hands and feet stay blueish gray.

Yep, he's in God's hands all right.

17 December 2008
Miracles

I almost forget to bring my pillow. Sarah holds it out to me at the last minute as I rush out the door, hop in the back of the Hiace and take a nap. In Kélo, we drop off André and his adopted daughter. They get on public transport bound for Léré.

Levi and I go to the TEAM mission station in Kélo to find some Arabic New Testaments. The rep for the Gideon's isn't there. I give him a call and he promises to meet me at noon at the Kélo hospital. I foolishly think I'll be done in Moundou before then.

An hour later we are in Moundou and go directly to the work site. Frederic, the construction boss, isn't there. I call him and while waiting check out the progress on the remodeling.

The back two rooms have been converted into one large room with three huge windows. A double door opens to the outside and a small door into the hallway. This will be the operating room. The trusses have been repaired, the roof replaced and the new ceiling mostly done.

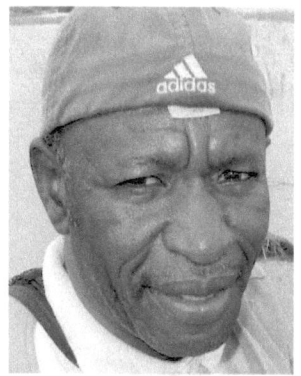

Anatole

I go back outside and see Anatole, our head lab tech in Béré. Two days ago I received a message that his son had meningitis here in Moundou.

"*Anatole, bonjour, ca va*? I tried to call you but I couldn't get through."

"Yeah, my phone was stolen at the hospital."

"I wanted to contact you to have you bring your son back to Béré, how did you find me here?"

"I just happened to see the Hiace drive by and followed it here."

Anatole explains how his son was treated. He started at the health center with once a day IM Quinine and Penicillin. When he didn't get better, the nurse referred him to the only hospital here in Moundou: the government operated Regional Medical Center.

The staff at the hospital started treatment for meningitis without doing any lab tests. The antibiotic prescribed, Ceftriaxone, wasn't available in the hospital pharmacy. Anatole had to purchase it on the black market for five times the price we get it for in Béré.

Nurses see the patients once a day, and only to give injections or perfusions. One day, the nurse came to give Anatole's son his shot. He prepared to inject with an empty, air-filled syringe. He didn't notice until Anatole pointed it out! In a week at the hospital, he saw a doctor once.

Last night, Anatole took him home. There at least he—Anatole himself —could make sure the meds were given when they were supposed to!

Antoine, the principal of the Adventist high school in Moundou shows up. Together we go to see the *Chef de Quartier* to find out about purchasing one or two of the empty lots next to our project. We bounce over the dirt streets of this industrial capital of Tchad and turn down a small side street before pulling up in front of a brick wall.

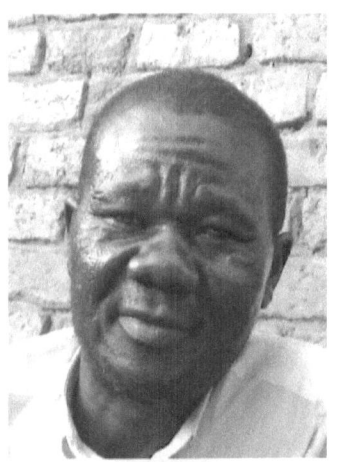

Antoine

Attached to the wall is a small lean to made of brick with a low ceiling out of tin. I stoop through the narrow door into a dark room filled with old men. The dim light comes through cracks in the bricks, ceiling and door illuminating several low wood slat chairs. In the middle is a rickety hand made coffee table with various documents spread across the top. The Chief is a wizened man in his late sixties or seventies with short, white curly hair and wearing a traditional long pocketed shirt and trousers. His right leg is wrapped in an elastic bandage.

The Chief motions us to some of the low chairs, only a few inches off the ground. I find myself basically squatting with the slats digging into my bony butt. Antoine starts speaking in Ngambai. I catch a few words like *docteur* and *hôpital*. After much dialogue, Antoine gives me the resume in French. The Chief knows the original owner of one lot and he'll ask who he sold it to. The owner of the second property is an old magistrate who has told the Chief to contact him if he finds a worthy buyer. He is very content that we're building a health institution in his neighborhood and will do all he can to help.

"It seems you are *malade,*" I speak to the chief in French, pointing to his leg. "Mind if I take a look?"

He motions for a young man outside who comes in. Between the two of us we lift up and unwrap the leg. There are a bunch of crumbled up dry leaves wrapped around the swollen ankle and foot: a typical traditional treatment for swelling. The other leg isn't swollen at all. I suspect early elephantiasis, prescribe him medicines for filarial worms and advise him to elevate his leg at night.

Just then, the pudgy old man to his right starts hacking. He's been coughing for several weeks. I prescribe him two antibiotics and an inhaler to open up his airways. I also let him know that if it doesn't get better in a week he should be tested for tuberculosis.

They are all very happy. The chief steps outside with us to wish us well and tell Antoine to check back tomorrow about the properties.

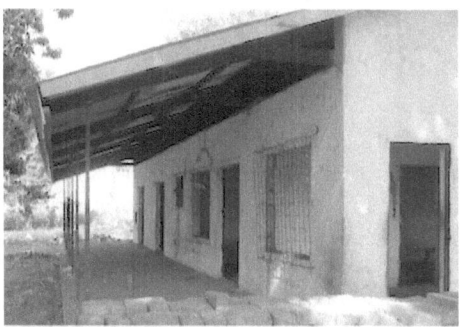

Progress Moundou Surgery Center

After running a few other errands, we stop at one of this metropolis's two gas stations. A couple of Arabs are lounging on chairs between the three antique pumps in the sandy courtyard. They slowly rise up as Levi places our three gas cans open in front of them and unlocks the gas tank.

I put my airplane fuel filter funnel in the tank opening as they warm up the pump. It slowly whirs into action and after a few minutes they start pumping. The gas spews in spurts and little bursts of air spraying the gasoline into our tank. After 18L it stops running.

"*Pardon, c'est fini*, that's the last of it. We should have some more tomorrow!"

Levi drives us to the second and last gas station. As we pull up the two guys sitting out front just look at us when we ask if they have gas and shake their fingers *"non"*.

We are forced to fuel up at the side of the road with gasoline from an old Cameroonian wine bottle. Then we pick up Anatole and his son who lays down in the back.

Levi drives us to Kélo without incident. The Post is closed. We go to the hospital. It's 2:00pm and Mathias, my contact for the Arab Bibles has gone home. We get his number from the nurse on night duty and he tells us to meet him at the Pili-Pili Hotel.

We pick him up, go back to the hospital to get the Bibles, and then return him directly to his house on the outskirts of town. As we head back towards the main road, a tall athletic man comes running after us in a green Arab robe barely covering his basketball shorts. He waves his hands and yells after us.

"You have a ton of packages at the Post Office. You need to pick them up tomorrow."

"We're heading back to Béré now and it's not an easy trip. We can't come back tomorrow. Can you open up the office and let us take them with us now?"

"*Ok! Ça va.*"

He hops in and we pick up 25 packages. Most are for the volunteers from their families, but one is for the hospital from the AMALF in France. It contains 150 vials of Ceftriaxone, an antibiotic we'd run out of and the exact one we need in order to treat Anatole's son's partially treated meningitis.

After we arrive in Béré, I pray with Anatole, convinced that God will heal his son. He has already intervened in so many small ways to bring us in contact and get us the exact medicine we need.

18 December 2008
Breech

As I burst through the door into the labor and delivery room, I suddenly realize how urgent the situation is.

I knew the woman in labor had a fetus in the breech position with one foot wanting to come out first. I'd told Hortence to alert me when she was completely dilated so I could assist the delivery.

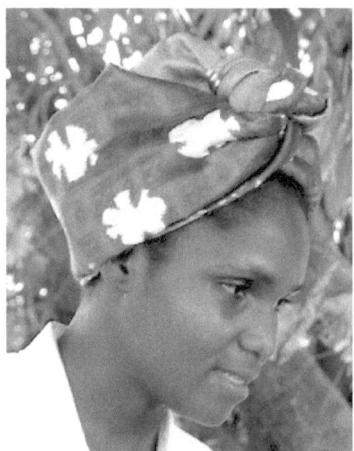

Hortence

Sarah came and told me that the woman was about to deliver so I wandered back over to the hospital. When I open the door, I size up the situation instantly and spring into action.

I see a woman lying on a metal table with her legs spread apart. Coming out of her is a small abdomen with two legs attached, flopping down onto the bed. No arms or head are visible. My first thought is to put on gloves. As I reach for the ones I'd washed and hung to dry earlier, I realize they are still too moist to get on quickly. I'm forced to work with my bare hands.

When the baby comes out feet first, it's very important that she deliver quickly. If not, the umbilical cord coming out of the abdomen will be compressed by the fetal head blocking off the blood circulation and its crucial supply of oxygen to the baby.

I have no time to lose since who knows how many minutes have flown by with the head stuck before I arrived.

I reach inside to try and free up the first arm. It won't budge. I twist the baby around so the other arm is on top. This time I'm able to hook it with my index finger and drag it down and out. I turn the baby over again and free up the other arm. Then I stick my finger in the baby's mouth and pull his chin down to his chest. I continue to tug with my other hand firmly grasping the baby's feet between my fingers.

The head pops out and the baby flops to the table. No tone. No cry. No breathing. Grayish blue color.

I quickly clamp and cut the cord. I move the limp mass over to the reanimation table. I start rapidly pressing the chest with one hand. I grab the bulb suction with the other to try and clear his airway. He has a faint, slow heartbeat.

I keep doing chest compressions. Hortence dries, stimulates and suctions the gunk out of the newborn's nostrils.

After what seems like hours, the heartbeat starts to pick up. The baby grimaces a little and seems like he wants to cough.

We continue our efforts.

Slowly but surely he starts to pink up. His heart rate becomes normal. But he's still pretty floppy and not breathing on his own.

Don't stop now, I tell myself.

Finally, his legs and arms start to curl up. He's getting some muscle tone and his body is now pink. At last, after I turn him over and give him a good whack on the back, he starts screaming like a banshee!

Two days later he is discharged home.

2009

30 January 2009

Niger

I am back in Africa after a month's holiday. Sarah, Gary and I have just flown eight hours across the desert from N'Djamena to Niamey, the capital of Niger. We cross dry grasslands, rocky outcroppings and fingers of the Sahara itching ever southward. Arriving over Niamey, we circle the Niger river and the new bridge being built by the Chinese before making a smooth landing at the airport.

As we taxi up, we see large men in black suits and dark glasses walking over to meet us. The President of the West African Division of Seventh-day Adventist, Gilbert Wari, Adventist Health International President Dick Hart, Dick's daughter Kari, and the Guptils are huddled together with Bill and Barbara Kirker in front of the VIP welcome center. Some of the men in black take our bags over on carts. Others whisk us through immigration and customs. Soon we are out front where black Mercedes and land cruisers wait with chauffeurs leaning casually against the front fenders.

Hazard lights flash as we make our way through the city ignoring lights and stop signs as other cars pull over to the side to let us pass. We arrive at the President's guest house overlooking the Niger River. Irrigated fields crowd the riverbanks. A sumptuous, yet simple supper awaits us. Air conditioned rooms, white table cloths, cold drinks and comfortable couches welcome us in style. Conversation flows easily as we are from time to time interrupted to meet more important people in dark suits.

The next morning starts with a tour. The ADRA director, Jason Brooks, takes us to their school where bright kids in sharp uniforms smile and shout out English phrases they have learned. The school is an impressive combination of underprivileged kids sponsored to go where they'd never have the opportunity to go otherwise, and rich kids who pay big to get a good education. All have become equals in their matching uniforms.

Next we have a rendezvous with the Nigerien President, Mamadou Tandja. Circling around the winding, well-guarded roads up to the governmental palace I feel it all is a little surreal. We climb up the massive steps and enter through a metal detector into an inner courtyard with high ceilings, traditional carved horses on stands, pictures and maps of Africa on the walls, and in the center a ten foot tall giraffe carved out of the twisted root system of a tree.

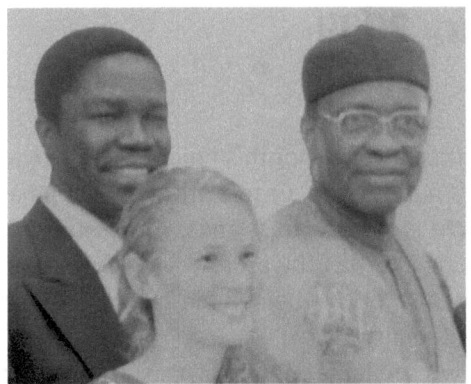

Gilbert, Sarah & Mamadou Tandja

After a few minutes, a distinguished man ushers us into the President's office. Bill Kirker introduces us as the group possibly willing to take on the management of the Mainé-Soroa Hospital. Mainé-Soroa just happens to be in the President's home town. I translate for Dick as he presents the President with a gift from Loma Linda University. The President is very gracious and poses for photos with all of us. On the spur of the moment, he gives Dick one of the carved horses in his lobby.

Whirlwind tours with more Mercedes, Land Cruisers and flashing lights take us to see various authorities: the Minister of Health turbaned in the Tuareg style, the distinguished Minister of Education with glasses perched on the tip of his nose, and the plump U.S. Ambassador.

The next day we start the 800km drive to Mainé-Soroa. It leads east across the desert towards Tchad. We make a quick stop at the only Christian hospital in Niger. We spend the night at the President's guest house half-way between Niamey and Mainé-Soroa. We crash on mattresses on the floor. All night long mice and mosquitos come for a closer look at the new visitors.

The next morning we hit the road for the last 600km to Mainé-Soroa. The second day's journey is uneventful except for two flat tires. On the outskirts of Mainé-Soroa, we stop at the side of the road in the middle of the desert. Our only companions are goats, sheep, donkeys, horses and camels meandering in between widely spaced scrub trees,.

As we get out of the cars on the outskirts of Mainé-Soroa, a crowd of people gathers around. Within minutes, the governor, the mayor, the prefect and a host of other dignitaries from the region arrive to welcome us. They then escort us into town to the king's quarters, in front of the central mosque next to the market.

A crowd has gathered. Brightly decorated horses mounted by robed, spear-and-sword-toting cavaliers prance on the sidelines. School kids in uniforms wave and chant. Turbaned, shirtless boys twist and contort in front of drum-pounding musicians beating out a fast rhythm accompanied by a bulging cheeked flute player. We push through the crowds to where chairs and couches have been arranged. The toothless, ninety-year old king nods and shakes hands as his eyes bulge out from behind coke-bottom glasses.

Important people give speeches. Kids dance, sing, shout and recite poems and slogans. Horsemen dress out and shake their weapons. Traditional dancers move and shake.

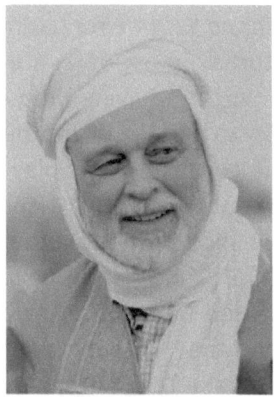

Dick as *Wokil*

At the end of the festivities, Dick is crowned *Wokil*. For the ceremony, Dick is brought crosslegged onto a mat in front of the king while the king's cronies circle around. They dress Dick in a traditional, blue robe with elaborate embroidery. Then they place a red, felt skull cap on his head and crown it with a turban. The *Wokil* is the king's new ambassador to the world, and in the absence of the king, his word is law. After the ceremonies, we go to Bill and Barbara's house for a feast of goat with couscous cooked in it's belly.

The next morning is another whirlwind tour. We first visit Barbara's Second Chance School. In Niger, children older than nine cannot start elementary school. This school is for those kids, to give them a chance at an education. We then go to the king's court and the Prefect's office in Mainé. Then it's on to Diffa to see the governor and back to Mainé to check out the ancient airstrip.

Friday morning we finally get to see the hospital which has been newly named the Kirker Hospital in honor of Bill and Barbara's efforts. Bill first came as a Peace Corps volunteer and then returned to be the only doctor around for years. He eventually founded a hospital in this extreme eastern city of Niger. Up til then the region had no functioning hospital.

After several years, Bill was forced to leave after a coup d'état destabilized the region. Within the last few years, Bill and Barbara were called back by President Tandja to revive the hospital.

The government is building new hospital wards and equipping the hospital. The Kirker Foundation has been managing the institution but Bill and Barbara are looking to retire so they've invited Adventist Health International (AHI) to help take over the management of the hospital.

Mindi Guptil is an Emergency Physician who grew up in Niger. Her and Scott are seriously considering coming to work at the Mainé Hospital if AHI decides to partner with the Kirker Foundation on this project.

Friday evening and Saturday, most of us are bedridden with vomiting and diarrhea. Saturday night, having mostly recovered, we are "fortunately" better enough to partake in another feast. This one is put on for the hospital staff and consists of a splayed roasted sheep and a couscous-filled goat. The goat is so tough I spend 15 minutes trying to chew a bite before I give up and spit it out in the toilet.

Sunday morning, Sarah, Dick, Kari and I head off in Bill's Land Cruiser across the desert. Dick refused Gary's offer to fly us back to Tchad. Dick wants to see Lake Tchad and the "famous" Lake Tchad cows. We head up north and around the top of Lake Tchad. It takes us thirteen hours to cross the desert into Tchad.

We see many camels, much sand, a few Lake Tchad thick-horned cows, one gazelle, one desert fox and a large bird whose name I forget. We pass clusters of white brick mud huts with flat roofs that have horns at the corners. We get stuck in the sand for at least half an hour. At the border we are cheerily welcomed. It seems we're the only car to have passed in two days. I consult one of the customs agents and prescribe antibiotics for his venereal disease. Finally, we arrive at the Tchadian town of Bol.

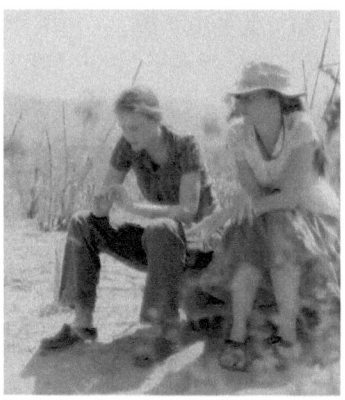

Sarah & Mindi

I am welcomed back to my host country by a couple of *moto-taxi* men trying to scam us into believing that the airport is a long ways away and only they can show us where it is. We ignore them and continue through the one road town to the hospital where the charge nurse on duty informs us that the *Nasara* we are looking for just landed his plane and is over at the regional medical officer's home. We soon find Gary accompanied by Noel, the Béré Hospital's chaplain.

The regional medical officer is a friend of Noel's. He welcomes us with a big smile and a feast of macaroni and tomato goat sauce. We partake of the food together, sitting on a mat with the tray of noodles in the middle. Everyone digs in with his own spoon and washes it down with bananas and cold water.

The next day, we fly off with Gary over the vast expanse of interconnected lakes which is what remains of the great Lake Tchad. Massive herds of cattle wander in long lines like ants across the green fields watered by what is still one of Africa's largest lakes only to end abruptly in the sands of the Sahel. After landing in Moundou and showing Dick and Kari the progress on our Surgery Center project there, we finally arrive back in Béré.

15 February 2009
Stuck

On my way to surgery, I pass by Augustin deep in conversation with the midwife Hortence. I briefly catch the words "breech presentation". I almost stop to ask what is going on. But ignoring my instinct, I continue on to the OR. I rationalize to myself that it must just be a prenatal visit or something. Certainly, they'll come and tell me if it's something serious.

Thirty minutes later, I'm calmly chatting with my friend and colleague Doug Wilson in the air-conditioned theater. Doug has come to volunteer with me for a couple weeks. We did Family Practice Residency together in Ventura County years ago. We are just finishing up a routine hernia operation. The external oblique is closed and we are preparing to close the skin. Doug and I have taken our time on the inguinal hernia repair, which I do with mosquito net mesh as usual.

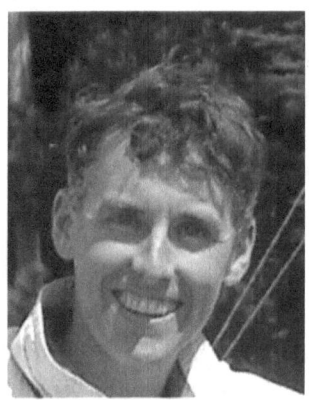

Doug

Suddenly, Hortence's head pops into the operating room through the swinging doors.

"There's a woman...the legs and body are out...the head's stuck...been that way for awhile...we can't..."

"I'm coming!" I cry "Doug, can you close up the skin?"

I strip off my surgical gown and bloody gloves. I race out through two sets of swinging doors, a screen door, around the corner, under the veranda, through another screen door and right into the tiny delivery room. I see a floppy set of legs and arms with no head plopped on the delivery table between a woman's blood-smeared spread legs. The room is packed with Augustin, Hortence, a mid-wife student, a new nurse named Prudence, Dr. Jacques, a family member and now myself.

I start to shout out orders.

"Augustin, get me the symphysiotomy kit! Hortence, bring me some gloves. Prudence, I need a syringe and some lidocaine. Jacques, a 20 blade scalpel."

As everyone goes off running I slip my hand inside the woman. A few futile tugs confirm that the baby's head, extended on it's neck, is stuck. Everyone is back in a matter of seconds. I slip on the gloves, draw up the lidocaine, open the instruments, inject quickly over the pubis, put the scalpel on the scalpel handle and speak directly to the woman.

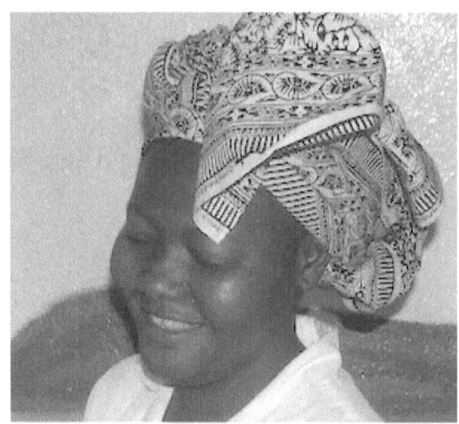

Prudence

"Don't move whatever you do if you want this to work! Augustin! Jacques! Grab her legs and pull them up and out!"

I slice through the skin and cartilage. The pelvis pops open. The baby slithers out. I clamp and cut the cord. I whisk him off to the exam table. He has no heartbeat, tone, movement, cry, respiration, color, nothing. I try and clear out the gunk in his mouth and nose. I do chest compressions for a couple minutes before silently covering him with a rag.

I turn my attention to the mother. I start to examine the position of the placenta and notice two things at once. First of all, her belly's still really big. Secondly, there's a bulging bag of water in her vagina. Twins!

I break the back of water and out pops a full head of hair. Within seconds the second twin is delivered, pulling up his arms and legs, grimacing and screaming his little lungs out.

He's alive!

23 February 2009
Congo

The never-ending, impregnable jungle finally gives way to the twisting silver snake of the river. My first view of the Congo is not as earth-shattering as I expected, but it is thrilling none the less. I am looking on that legendary waterway immortalized in so many writings that feeds central Africa with its numerous tributaries and irresistible tug towards the ocean.

I am crammed tight in the left rear seat of a Cessna 172. Gary and Jeremy have flown me straight from Béré down to Moundou, across Central African Republic and finally into the Democratic Republic of Congo where I get my first glimpse of its mighty river. There is a water jug between my feet. Provisions stacked to the ceiling next to me force me to curl up almost in the fetal position. My only relief is to turn from my right side to my left occasionally. To pass the time I immerse myself deep into the book *Seabiscuit*.

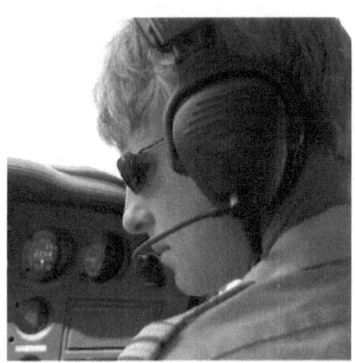

Jeremy

We begin our descent across the Congo River and land at the tiny airport of Kisangani. The immigration officials look fierce and determined to shake down these foreigners for some "tea money" until Gary starts speaking to them in Swahili. He explains that he grew up in Eastern Zaire as DRC was known back then. We then have no problems with the authorities who are fascinated by this white African. Outside, Keith Mosier is waiting to take us to the Congo Frontline Mission compound.

Over meals rich in pineapple, bananas and avocados, we hear about the Mosiers' efforts. They want to start a medical mission program to meet the medical needs of the outlying villages. For now, a simple canoe with an outboard motor and a local doc takes them a few miles outside of town to provide basic malaria, malnutrition and parasite treatments. As they've come face to face with burn victims, people maimed for life through various accidents and the incredible infant mortality rates, they realize that much more needs to be done.

As the stories unfold around me, I am taken back to the three and a half months I spent on the Amazon River working with the *Luzeiro* mission launch program back in 1994. I remember reading the stories of Leo Halliwell and his wife as they opened up the Amazon basin with their little medical launch and handfuls of quinine for malaria. As I mention this out loud, Keith walks over to the bookshelf and pulls out a book, *Light in the Jungle*. I'd read it 15 years ago, but am ready to read it again.

I start reading that very night as deep longings I had buried inside over the years start to be awakened. The river is calling me.

The next day Gary and I go to help Keith and his dad try and negotiate with the Ministry of Public Works. They want to rent a bulldozer to clear the jungle from the land they want to build their school on. Things are rough for a while and negotiations tense. Finally, I mention that I am a doctor and we are interested in opening a medical river boat program.

Suddenly, the scowling Minister stands up and stretches out his hand with a big smile on his face.

"I'm a surgeon too. I've operated on everything. Welcome, colleague. If you ever need any papers or authorizations to get this project through to the right people, just bring it to me and I'll accelerate it right through."

The next morning, Gary, Jeremy and I fly Brazzaville. There we happen to meet up with Gilbert Wari again. He is accompanied by Rosa Banks, one of the under secretaries of the General Conference of Seventh-day Adventists. As we are given the tour of the mission compound, we come across a map of Congo.

There, again, the River jumps out at me.

Running all the way up the border between Congo and the Democratic Republic of Congo (DRC) it then branches off into the interior of DRC. However, another major tributary continues up the border until it reaches Bangui, the capital of Central African Republic (CAR). The River then curves eastward across the border of CAR and DRC. Hundreds of smaller tributaries pour into the River from the Congo side making it possible to reach most of the abandoned little villages with a medical launch.

Sunday, I finally get to touch the Congo River. We have somehow managed to get all the stamps and pay all the fees to cross from Brazzaville to Kinshasa. Nowhere else in the world are two country capitols this close. We climb in the boat and the captain starts up the motor. We weave our way through a slalom course of grass and reed floaters scattered across the breadth of our course. I dip my hand into the cool water and lean back to inhale the smell of the River and absorb the majesty of its greatness.

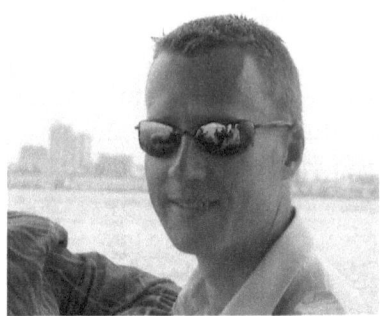

Gary & Kinshasa

We are given a tour of Kinshasa by the honorable Bahati, a member of the House of Representatives. He first takes us to the Adventist mission station. Years ago, the church had built a hospital boat that never got off the ground thanks to the Congo civil war. It was finally sold for a pittance in 2003. We wanted to find out what happened to it.

The president of the mission escorts us up to his office. He spreads out on his desk a wad of pictures of the boat under construction and the all-but-finished product. It is almost exactly what I'd been imagining and looks remarkably similar to the boats I'd worked on in Brazil.

The next morning our Hewa Bora flight takes off from Kinshasa bound for Lubambashi. The early morning sun casts a warm glow across the River as it spreads out in a flood plane filed with islands above the falls downriver.

It is beckoning...

25 February 2009
Lubambashi

The plane has stopped. I thought we were going directly to Lubambashi. Suddenly, we find ourselves on the ground at another airport. I see people getting up and climbing down the stairs that open up from the tail of the old 727 airplane. I was actually extremely cold during the flight. I decide to take a breath of warm Congolese air outside. A sharply dressed young Congolese man is standing at the foot of the stairs just under the middle engine. We strike up an easy conversation until he notices something dripping on his suit.

At first, I think it is fuel. On closer inspection, it turns out to be simply water. The man is very friendly. I explain that we are with Adventist Medical Aviation and are doing some research on the possibilities of doing medical work on the Congo River.

At this point our attention is caught by a large mobile staircase being pushed past us to the right engine of the plane a few feet away. Some men scramble up to the engine and start taking off the bottom enclosure. As jet fuel starts to cascade out, the ground crew rushes around collecting plastic buckets to catch it in. A small puddle forms and flows off the runway.

A man in a suit rambles up lugging an ancient, twisted metal tool chest. He folds it out from the middle into several trays carrying some large, simple tools. He selects a large screwdriver and climbs up the ladder to the now-exposed engine as a couple of blue-overall wearing maintenance guys scrape out the fuel left in the bottom of the casing.

The mechanic tinkers around and eventually manages to pull off what appears to be the fuel filter. He takes off the filter and examines the cover which appears to be missing a gasket. He shows it around to a few other people amidst the shaking of heads and then puts it right back on. He tightens it up well. The blue guys mop up the remaining jet fuel with rags. Meanwhile, more ground crew have sloshed the tarmac underneath the engine with buckets of sudsy water.

The mechanic puts the engine cover back on. The flight attendant ushers us back up the stairway into the plane. We take off and miraculously land again at Lubambashi without further incident

.A thin, light skinned man with a huge smile, blue ringed brown eyes and a warm handshake greets us at immigration along with a short, stocky dark man who speaks some decent English. We breeze through passport control and are taken to the Adventist Surgery and Gynecology Clinic in a Toyota Hilux. The Hilux Surfs are everywhere, but unfortunately, no boards or waves are to be seen anywhere.

Most of the vehicles in town have the steering wheel on the right side of the car. This is strange, since they also drive on the right. It seems most of the cars are imported from British East Africa where they drive on the left.

We arrive at the clinic and are told there is an emergency. They are just waiting for the surgeon, Dr. Delgado to arrive.

When I inform them I'd like to assist, they drag me up some steep winding stairs to the attic which serves as pharmacy and stock room. I'm given a pair of elastic waist band scrubs and slippers too small for my feet. I quickly change, go downstairs and enter the operating room.

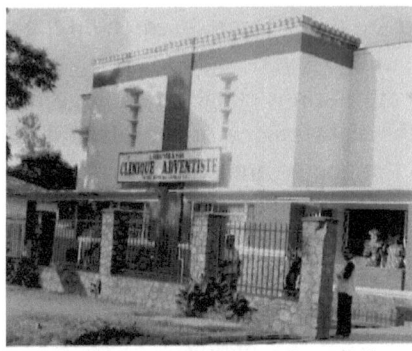

Lumbambashi Adventist Clinic

The OR is small and long with tile running from floor to ceiling. X-rays showing obvious bowel obstruction are illuminated on a viewer straight ahead over the operating table. On the table, covered in a hospital gown is a young 14 year old girl with a nasogastric tube coming out of her nose attached to an old IV bottle for gastric drainage.

At the foot of the table is a metal tray covered with a dark green cloth filled with shiny instruments. The surgical assistant presides over everything robed from head to foot in the same dark green. His white surgical gloves rapidly arrange the instruments guided by his eyes half hidden behind a blue mask and protective goggles.

At the head of the bed is a jolly, pudgy man in ill-fitting scrubs whose large smile can't be contained by that silly piece of paper trying to pose as a surgical mask. In answer to my inquiries he shows me his anesthesia setup.

The archaic monitor is black and green with erratic QRS complexes running together on the EKG lead making their form, rate and rhythm almost impossible to interpret. But that is child's play next to trying to read the blood pressure and heart rate which for some reason are projected as mirror images of themselves.

The anesthesia machine consists of a metal table with bars on the back. An oxygen extractor behind the machine runs a rigged tubing apparatus up to a canister attached to the bar. The inhaled anesthetic is put in the canister and regulated with a twisting knob that the anesthetist proudly says he made himself. He shows me the scoring marks on the knob that let him roughly know the concentration given.

Laid out in an orderly fashion on the table are four endotracheal tubes, a laryngoscope and three unmarked syringes containing, according to him, Valium/Atropine, Thiopental and Succinylcholine.

Just then, Dr. Delgado bursts into the room. An Argentinean of Peruvian descent, Delgado has been in DRC for over 20 years. He started at the Songa Adventist Hospital before moving to Lubambashi and opening this surgery and gynecology center. He is known all over the region as the best surgeon around, is personal friends with the governor, has performed over 12,000 major operations there and has trained countless young Congolese physicians and medical students in the art of surgery.

But I was to learn all that later. For the moment, Delgado is focused on the task at hand.

"What's her story?" He asks the resident who called him in.

"She was sick since Friday, went into another clinic on Saturday, was given malaria treatment and sent off for a bunch of lab tests and x-rays. After three days, she was getting worse and the family brought her here. When we examined her, she had an acute abdomen with signs of obstruction. As soon as we told the family she needed an operation, they wanted to evacuate her to South Africa until we assured them you would come yourself and do the operation."

"Ok, well she obviously needs surgery, it's too bad they waited. I'll go scrub."

Soon the operation is under way. On entering the abdominal cavity, we find pus everywhere with the small intestines stuck together. It takes awhile to clean things up and separate out the intestines to find just what we suspected, a perforated appendicitis.

After the appendectomy, massive irrigation and placement of a drain, Delgado leaves the closure to the residents. As the residents work, Delgado tells me about his latest project: a new surgery hospital on the outskirts of town.

The anesthetist extubates the girl and she is wheeled off to post-op recovery in stable condition.

That evening, I check up on our young patient. She is lying comfortably with no fever and only slight tachycardia. Her abdomen is still slightly swollen, but soft and I already hear a few bowel sounds. I talk with the father who is eternally grateful. He tells me that his son has just returned from a visit to Orlando, Florida where my parents live. His daughter wants to go there for nursing school.

As he gives me a ride back to the Union offices where I'm staying, I offer to put him in contact with the SDA nursing school at Florida Hospital. He likes the idea and takes my email address. He insists we come eat at his restaurant the next day, but unfortunately, we already have plans.

The last day before heading back to Kinshasa, I make my final rounds and find the girl in even better condition. She's already passed gas letting us know that bowel function is returning. I pray with the family one more time and leave.

13 March 2009
Ostomy

"Doctor, you need to see this baby," Samedi calls me to the ER. "She's only seven days old, but she's never had a bowel movement."

I pull back the curtain around the ER bed and see a frightened mother holding her newborn baby in her arms. The infant's belly is markedly distended, but still somewhat soft. I listen and hear good bowel sounds. The mother says she breastfeeds well and goes on to prove it by feeding the baby right in front of me. I examine the perineum and the anus is present.

"Samedi, could you get me a glove and some lubricant?"

He comes back in a few minutes. I slip the glove on my right hand, apply some goo and gently press my pinky into the tiny anus. I slowly dilate it until my finger can go all the way in. It's a blind rectal pouch as I suspected.

"The girl will need surgery immediately," I inform the parents. They agree.

Without an x-ray, I'm forced to guess exactly the extent of the malformation of the colon. I'm hoping it's just the sigmoid (the last part of the large intestine) that's not open. Sarah and Siméon tag team the anesthesia calculating the tiny doses of Atropine and Ketamine for it's small, 2.4 kg frame. We strap her onto the Papoose board so she can't move. Abel preps her distended abdomen with Betadine. Then he and I scrub, drape the belly and pray before cutting.

I decide to gamble that I can make a colostomy from the descending colon. I cut a small circle out of her skin to the left of her bellybutton, cut through the fascia and muscles and enter the peritoneal cavity. Small intestines burst out under pressure and I can't get them back in. I move to the center and make a midline incision releasing the pile of intestines to the outside air. I then bring back those that have gone out the side hole and explore inside. The colon hasn't formed (atresia) all the way from beginning to end. The whole thing looks like a long appendix running from cecum to rectum.

Everything is so tiny. I take a part of the ileum about 10 cm from where it joins the cecum and clamp the bowel with non-crushing clamps. I divide the intestine and slowly identify the miniscule vessels in the mesentery and clamp, cut and tie them. I open up the distal end, suction out all the meconium resting there and suture it closed in two layers.

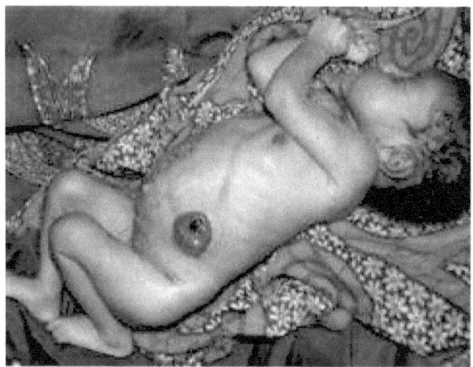

Baby with ostomy

I pull out the proximal part through the side window, sew the wall to the strong fascia, evert the gooey mucosa and suture that to the skin. I then suck out all the stool from nine months in mommy and seven days in the real world. Finally, I close up the midline incision after irrigating the abdomen profusely.

I write post-op antibiotic and immediate breastfeeding orders and go home. Except for needing malaria treatment with rectal quinine, she has a routine post-op course. She will have her sutures removed in a few days.

15 March 2009
The Bell Tolls

It's early Sunday morning and the drums are pounding: deep, holding bass thumps with rhythmic higher pitched hypnotizing beats wafting through the background. In a few minutes, a mournful call pierces the African pre-dawn calling the faithful to the first prayer of the day:

"Allaaaaaaaaaah-hu akbar! Allaaaaaaa-aaaah-hu akbarrrrr!"

Finally, to complete the symphony, church bells start tolling across town as the dawn breaks. But the music is rudely interrupted by a harsh clanging on our sheet metal door that can only be pounded out by the bare knuckles of a nurse seeking a doctor.

"*Oui*?!" I mumble.

"*C'est moi, Augustin.*"

"I'm coming!"

I fumble for my shorts hanging over the foot of the bed and stumble out the door to the porch. I open the screen door and come face to face with our charge nurse. He's carrying a flashlight and a small *carnet* which serves as a patient's portable medical record.

"I just received a young boy who has respiratory distress. His whole chest caves in and you can hear the noise of his breathing clear across campus."

I hurriedly put on my scrubs and follow Augustin through the bushes, around Lazare's fire pit, under the mango trees, on top of the straw and horse poop, to the side of the container, and through the gate into the hospital compound. I understand what Augustin means as I hear a high pitched rasping coming from the dimly lit emergency room door.

A young boy is slouched across his mother's lap as she balances on a stool. She holds him up under the arm pits as his lower chest literally caves in all the way to his spine. He is desperately trying to suck in oxygen as he lets out a stridorous breath. His eyes bug out and almost roll back in his head. I listen to his chest with my stethoscope and hear practically nothing. I place it on his neck and hear loud stridor. I get him to open his mouth and where the back of his throat should be is a smooth, bulging mass.

I'm afraid I won't get him to the operating room in time. I call our new volunteer nurse, Caroline, to help me and pick up the child in my arms. I jog over to the operating room, flip the padlock to the secret code, insert the key in the door and burst into the operating room. Fortunately, this morning the batteries have held their charge through the night and we have light. However, I'm afraid the power will go out any minute. I send Augustin to wake up Steve to turn on the generator.

Meanwhile, I lay the child on the operating table and give him a shot of IM Ketamine. Caroline searches for an IV. Just then, power goes out...

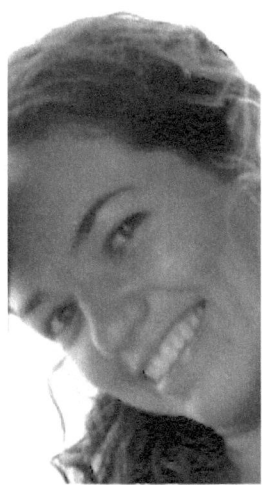

Caroline

Within seconds, though, I hear the slowly increasing "thump thump thump" of the Lister engine starting up. In a few more seconds I can turn on the overhead operating room lights and we are back in business.

I dump the cardboard box of endotracheal tubes on the floor. I rifle through them searching for one small enough for my patient. I finally find a 6.0 un-cuffed tube. I grab the laryngoscope out of the bottom drawer of the anesthesia machine as I slip on gloves.

Caroline now has the IV running and the Ketamine is working. His oxygen saturation is 35%. I find a guide wire, put it in the ET tube, check the light on the laryngoscope, raise the bed and open the kid's mouth. There is no way I'm going to see the vocal cords, the entire back of the throat is swollen shut.

I toss the equipment aside. I grab a 15 blade scalpel and a suture removal kit. I slice vertically down the middle of the neck, find the space between the tracheal and cricoid cartilages and poke through into his wind pipe with a hemostat. I spread it open, suction out blood and shove in the ET tube.

I then hook up an Ambu bag and give him some breaths. The chest rises and I see vapor in the tube. I check with a stethoscope hear breath sounds only on the right. The tube's in too far. I pull it out slightly and listen again to confirm there's now bilateral breath sounds. I suture the wound closed with the tube in place. Caroline continues bagging.

His oxygen saturation is now up to 92%. I stop bagging and just let him breath through the tube. His sats hover around 84-88% which isn't great. However, we don't have a ventilator or adequate lab tests so it's more dangerous to bag him then to let him breath on his own.

I then try to place a nasogastric tube so he can be fed past the obstruction in his throat. It won't pass. I stick my finger in his mouth and try to shove the tube in through his nose while feeding it past the mass with my finger. Suddenly, pus gushes out his mouth. I've ruptured the peritonsillar abscess. I quickly suck out the foul smelling pus and am relieved that it was so easily taken care of.

Caroline and I wheel him out to his room and give his family instructions.

Later that evening, I go to check on him and find his tube choked up with secretions. All we have to suck it out with is a newborn suction device. It allows me to put one end down the ET tube and then by sucking on the other end pull out the gunk into a chamber between the two ends. Very high tech. He starts to breath easier. I ask Jason to check on him every hour and suction as needed.

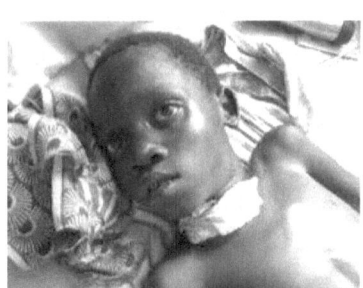

Boy with trach

The next morning, he is awake, but tired. He is breathing fairly easily through the tube. I have the family members sit him up. I suction him one more time even though the tube is pretty clear. I move on to the other hospitalized patients.

In less than 15 minutes, Annie comes running up to me and says breathlessly, "Stuff's coming out his trach, he's not breathing!"

I run back to his room and see instantly his tube is clogged up with pus that's dripping out. As I grab the suction to clear his airway, I see he's not breathing. His eyes are rolled back in his head. He has no pulse. As I suction, Jacques starts chest compressions. When the airway is clear I attach the bag and start breathing for him.

We take him to the operating room quickly. We attach our cardiac monitor. He finally gets a heartbeat back with a pulse. But after a few minutes it slows down again until we do more chest compressions to bring it back up. We try multiple doses of Atropine and Adrenaline. His oxygen saturation stays in the mid to upper 80's when we bag him.

But he just doesn't want to come back. Finally, after 90 minutes we are forced to stop. We wrap him in a cloth and call in the family. The dad nods, he's been expecting it. He wraps the boy up in his arms, carries him out and the family mournfully walks out the gate.

The drum beats on. The call to prayer continues. The bell keeps on tolling.

21 March 2009
HELLP

I start rounds right across from labor and delivery. I discharge a tall man I'd operated on two days ago for hydrocele and hernia. Before leaving, I advise him to stop drinking as his alcoholism made his Ketamine anesthesia difficult.

Next is a pregnant woman who came in yesterday with a hemoglobin of 4.3 g/dl. She sits with a blood bag attached to her arm with the plasma still inside. She has got two 450ml bags of whole blood. She needs more, but no family members can be found.

The baby with the ileostomy is sleeping comfortably beside her mother. The ostomy that herniated out last night is back in place and the midline incision appears to be healing well.

The little girl in the old maintenance closet turned into isolation ward is sitting up half naked eating some porridge. Six days of Chloramphenicol with a single dose of Ceftriaxone have done wonders to transform her meningitis coma into the hope of full recovery.

Moving past the nurses station and the chaplain's office, I greet a Fulani nomad woman. She has a long wound sewn up across her chest into her armpit like a gunnysack. She had a massive breast tumor that went into her axillary lymph nodes. The deep cavity left by the removed lymph nodes has become infected and is being dressed with diluted bleach. She wants to go back to the bush where she can drink milk from her own cows. She just doesn't like the food available here in Béré. We finally convince her son that she should stay until the wound is healed.

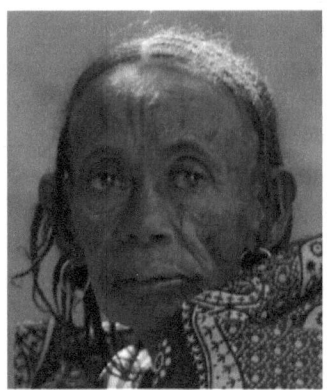

Fulani woman

Two men operated on yesterday for large inguinal scrotal hernias grace the next two beds. I have the nurses take out the IVs and tell them to get up and start moving to avoid post-op complications.

Beside them is a woman who's life we barely saved three months ago. She had been in labor for three days. She came in with a decomposing baby stuck in her small pelvis. A symphysiotomy brought the baby out quickly. However, the gangrenous perineal flesh had to be debrided several times. Then we packed her vagina for weeks with diluted bleach soaked compresses and gave her heavy doses of antibiotics. As a result of the prolonged labor, she developed an enormous vesicle-vaginal fistula and a scarred down vaginal vault and cervix.

Three days ago I attempted a vaginal repair with not much success. That evening I was awoken by a sense of God's presence. An idea came to me on how to help her. The next day I opened up her bladder from the abdominal side. I inserted a ureteral catheter into her right ureter to drain the urine out the abdominal wall. Her left ureter appeared scarred down and the catheter wouldn't pass. I then closed up the vesicle-vaginal fistula from inside the bladder. I left a foley catheter in the urethra and the ureteral catheter I brought out through her lower abdominal wall.

Today there is clear urine out of the right ureteral catheter and bloody urine out of the bladder drain. That means maybe her left ureter is working after all. More importantly, she has no vaginal leakage.

An emaciated Arab lies across the way. I saw him at 4:30am. He had almost no blood pressure and a raging fever. He responded to IV fluids and IV quinine. I suspect he has AIDS. I put him on broad spectrum antibiotics. His HIV status is confirmed later and he dies in the early afternoon.

Meanwhile I move on to the middle aged woman who had a hysterectomy yesterday for fibromas. She is doing well. Next to her is a woman who has had her knees permanently bent since the age of 12 due to burn contractures until January when Dr. Bond released her right leg. I released her left leg in February and the wounds are healing well. She can almost straighten both legs now.

First bed on the left in the men's ward is a man with an abscess deep in his thigh to the side of his hip joint and back into his gluteus. The drain I placed when I drained the pus is still working. The swelling and pain have gone down.

His neighbor is another patient operated on for a hernia. I discharge him as well. To the right is a man with gangrene of the scrotum. I debrided him six days ago. Yesterday, we found he had malaria and a hemoglobin of 4.7 g/dl. He is still waiting for other family members to come. None of the ones tested yesterday has the right blood type. His wound is much better, though, and he is sitting up comfortably.

Next are the two miracle burn kids. They are almost healed despite our being unable to give them skin grafts because of lack of equipment. Little Bai has become Sarah's adopted son. He walks around with her squirting patients with syringes full of water and sitting in her lap for morning worship. The older girl is healing well but is depressed and doesn't want to get up.

The next young man was stabbed clear through the front of his shin between his two leg bones into the back of his calf. He came in days later with a very swollen lower leg. I thought he had an abscess. I took him to the operating room by myself. When I incised the "abscess" instead of pus I found myself removing massive clumps of blood clot.

Suddenly, there was a surge of pent up, raging blood. Since it was coming from behind the tibia there was no way to compress it. I ran and pulled out a used suction tubing from a basin. I quickly tied it around his leg above the knee to stop the bleeding before calling in help. Once Siméon, Abel and Caroline arrived, we opened up his calf, dissected down to the vessels, sutured the hole in the artery and tied off both ends of the vein.

Today, he complains of foot pain. I prescribe Ibuprofen and paracetamol.

His neighbor is a man who we initially saw two months ago for an open tibia fracture. He refused treatment at the time. A month later, he came back. His leg was completely infected, swollen, edematous and spilling out pus from the fracture site. Needless to say, the bones had not healed.

We had to radically remove the front of the tibia. Then we pierced his tibia with four Steinmann pins attached to some PVC pipe to act as an external fixator. The wound still smells, but is improving. Fortunately, the pus around the pins is starting to dry up.

Now that rounds are finishing, I tell Siméon and Abel to go ahead and prepare the woman for the hysterectomy, do the spinal anesthesia and call me when they're ready. Meanwhile I round on a pediatric ward filled with malaria kids, most of whom are recovering and can be sent home.

I do the fastest hysterectomy of my life and go out to do a couple of ultrasounds while the operating room crew prepares a four year old boy with bladder stones. As I approach my office a well-dressed woman greets me with her cute little daughter. The girl is about four years old. She is wearing a spotless, frilly, baby blue dress, has newly braided hair and sports a sweet smile as she proffers me her hand in a shy greeting.

"Do you recognize her?" the mom asks. "You delivered her by C-section in 2004 when you first came here."

I don't remember, but smile and nod. I go into my office with a warm feeling in my heart. I finish the first ultrasound and Sarah peeps in the door.

"You better see this patient in the ER."

"You mean now? Is it urgent?"

"Yes, this woman is crashing!"

I rush out across the courtyard, under the mango trees and into the ER. A woman lies on an army stretcher barely breathing. Her eyes are swollen shut and she's gurgling with a weak respiratory effort. She is obviously pregnant.

"Augustin, Prudence! Can you help? Grab her and bring her directly to the operating room!"

We dump her directly onto the operating room table. I prepare to intubate her. Abel quickly finds an IV. She starts to bleed. I search for her vocal cords in vain. Everything is swollen. I finally slip the ET tube through with help from Siméon's cricoid pressure.

"Let's get another IV going!" I tell Abel. "Siméon, check her hemoglobin and blood sugar!"

Her body is burning with fever. We have Ringer's Lactate running wide open on her right arm and IV quinine on her left. Siméon has put in an nasogastric tube. Nasty gastric contents spill onto the floor from the open urine bag attached to the end of the tube. She starts to gurgle blood from her nose and mouth in frothy spurts. Siméon suctions. Results are back: she has severe hypoglycemia.

"Sarah, get some glucose running, quick!"

I go get the ultrasound from my office. I confirm a normal fetal heartbeat, cephalic presentation and 33 weeks estimated gestational age. Her blood pressure is initially normal but suddenly skyrockets and stays high. We do a urine dipstick which is highly positive for protein suggesting a diagnosis of pre-eclampsia. With her enlarged liver and uncontrollable bleeding I also suspect HELLP syndrome. The only thing is to deliver the baby.

C-section baby

A quick, uneventful C-section brings a small, but well-developed boy into the world. He has great tone and is grimacing. I pass him off to Hortence and turn back to the woman. I sew up the uterus, fascia and skin. The woman is still doing poorly with heart rate over 150/minute, high blood pressure and low O2 saturation. Blood is everywhere as she continues to spray bloody foam all over.

I don't hear a cry from the baby. Hortence said earlier he was breathing. I go over to look and find him pale, limp, with no respiratory effort and a slow heartbeat. I am furious! I desperately do CPR to try and bring him back, but it's too late.

We leave the woman in the operating room on a gurney where we can monitor and suction her. Siméon hangs up two bags of whole blood. We hope the platelets will help stop the bleeding.

We operate on the four year old pulling out two marble sized stones. At the end of the case, the woman is still breathing but her sats are in the low 80's. The watery blood continues to well up out of her nostrils and gurgle out her oral airway. We had to take out her ET tube since we don't have a ventilator.

I quickly repair an inguinal hernia on a female patient. When I'm done, we decide to just wheel the woman with HELLP syndrome out to the wards. The family is getting anxious and people don't understand when someone dies in the operating room. They tend to think you killed them.

Gasps of fear flutter up from the crowd of relatives gathered outside surgery as we wheel the blood specked woman and gurney out to the wards. We drop her in a bed and I tell the husband to wipe up the blood as it spouts out of the mouth and nose. I write orders for IV fluids and IV quinine.

I move on.

06 June 2009
Drought

I feel a cold sweat creeping along the surface of my skin. A sensation of nausea rises to my throat. I desperately try to focus my eyes somewhere that will calm the waves of motion sickness. The Cessna 172 lurches and plunges in the turbulence 7500 feet above the surface of the desert in a wall of dust and clouds. There is no escape.

"I think I might need one of those barf bags Sarah just brought you." I stoically mention to Gary.

"Here, you better start flying again," offers Gary. "That often helps. It gives you a little sense of control when it's turbulent."

I grab the controls and try to remember to make small adjustments back and forth and side to side as my gaze shifts rapidly between the horizon and the various instruments on the panel. I try to maintain altitude, direction, vertical speed, and bearings as the thermals rising from the hot sand below buffet us up and down and side to side.

My nausea slowly disappears.

An hour later as we approach Béré, I give the controls back to Gary for the landing. The two men in the back from the Tchadian government who have come to evaluate our work at the hospital break the silence with a heartfelt *"Dieu merci"* as the plane touches down smoothly and taxis in to the waiting hospital van.

I greet Levi warmly as we pack up and head to the hospital. What was starting to turn green with the early April rains has changed to a dreary brown.

"I guess I must have taken the rain with me to the U.S.," I joke with Levi. "A week after arriving in Florida they had a two week long rain storm that ended their drought. Don't worry, though, I brought it back with me!"

We both laugh, but half hope it's true. People are already starting to talk about famine this year (although they do so every year no matter how much rain we get).

I get our visitors settled in the guest house and change into scrubs to take a quick tour of the hospitalized patients.

The Arab man with the broken tibia and jaw is elated to see me and immediately asks to have the PVC pipe external fixator removed. The wiring on his jaw was taken off a few days ago. His mandible seems to be well healed. The leg looks good too. We'll have to send him to Moundou for an x-ray since ours has been broken for years.

Mathieu, the other man with a PVC pipe external fixator, waves to me from across the room. I greet him and take a brief look at the wound. It has closed up some, but is still quite deep where I removed the infected bone.

That evening I am woken up by a fierce wind followed by scattered rains. The next few days we have several intense thunderstorms.

The drought is over.

10 June 2009 AM
Kaleb

"Hurry to the ER, James! Run!" The familiar words come not in the usual African French but in the familiar English of our friends, Gary and Wendy Roberts, as they whiz by the house on their motorcycle.

I'd gotten up a little before 5:00am. I'm writing email when I hear the roar of the *moto* and the cries of the anguished parents. I quickly pull on some scrubs and rush out the door where I run into Sarah who's just come to get me. She is just finishing up a night shift in the ER. It's about 6:00am.

The hospital is bathed with an early morning tranquility that would've been soothing on any other morning but this one. I arrive at the ER and see Gary bent over his son, Kaleb, giving him mouth to mouth resuscitation. Kaleb's pale, limp body seems to want to sink into the top of the desk he's lying on.

"He was still breathing as we were coming," cries Gary. "But he just stopped. He has no heart beat!"

I start giving chest compressions as I bark out orders to Sarah, Wendy, Koumabas, Hortence and Augustin who fortunately happen to be there.

"Get some IV glucose and some IV tubing! Someone find an IV! Call the lab for a hemoglobin and glucose check! Get the pulse ox from the operating room!"

As they rush off to find the material, I look closer at Kaleb. His body is flaccid, face is pale and haggard, eyes are closed, mouth is half open and a mild gurgling comes out of his throat with each chest compression. He has no heart beat and his lungs sound filled with fluid. His belly is soft with an enlarged liver.

Gary takes over chest compressions as Hortence hands me the D5W attached to some IV tubing. I attach the tubing to a butterfly needle and insert it under the skin of his stomach for a subcutaneous perfusion of glucose. His blood sugar may be low.

"Hortence, give him half an ampoule of IV furosemide IM."

Augustin is patiently searching for an IV on Kaleb's small, white hands and arms. Sarah arrives with the pulse oximeter. We continue chest compressions. The O2 sat is 15%. I have Gary start rescue breathing again. The pulse ox stops working.

"Sarah, get some Adrenaline and Atropine from the operating room!"

Still no IV.

"Koumabas, get me a blue IV catheter and a 5mL syringe!"

Gary does two rescue breaths for every ten of my chest compressions. Wendy has come back with an epi-pen and accidentally sticks her thumb with it instead of Kaleb's leg.

Sarah gives Adrenaline and Atropine intramuscularly.

I listen and detect a faint, slow heart beat. We continue CPR.

"Wendy, find me one of those small red, urine catheters in the operating room so we can empty his bladder!"

Koumabas gives me the IV catheter with which I miraculously find his right femoral vein on the first try despite feeling no pulse and am able to thread the catheter in. I attach the IV glucose bottle and let it run in.

Meanwhile Mathieu has arrived and now has the results: hemoglobin a little low and blood sugar extremely low.

Wendy returns with the foley and Augustin drains Kaleb's bladder. Kaleb's lungs are clearer. He still has a faint heartbeat.

"Sarah, inject the Adrenaline as rapidly as you can....now!" I quickly pump Kaleb's heart has fast as I can with my external compressions to get the medicine to his heart.

"Sarah, take over chest compressions, I'm going to fnd some Magnesium in my office!"

The magnesium goes in the IV fluids and slowly trickles in. Gary still does rescue breathing. Wendy offers to take over but Gary wants to keep going.

"Mathieu, can we do a Potassium?"

"*Oui!*"

I draw a milliliter of dark blood from Kaleb's femoral vein and Mathieu hurries off to the lab.

CPR continues. We've been going for 40 minutes. I listen to Kaleb's chest. No heartbeat. We continue CPR.

"Sarah, more atropine."

Gary speaks up after his two rescue breaths. "Should we stop?"

"Let's go just a little more," I reply.

Atropine is in.

We continue CPR for five more minutes.

I listen to Kaleb's heart...

Nothing.

We stop.

Gary and Wendy collapse weeping into each others arms as sobs explode from within my chest. I grab Gary from the side my arm draped across his neck. Sarah is on the other side hugging Wendy.

Gary solemnly wraps up the still, little body.

"Do you want to use the van?" I ask. "We can drive you back home."

Gary turns to Wendy, "No, let's just put him between us on the motorcycle and take him home."

"Anything we can do?"

"No, we just want some alone time. Then in the afternoon we'll have a service." They trudge out to the motorcycle, the quiet bundle in Gary's arms.

Tears streaming down my face, I walk slowly back home. I think back to September 3, 2001 when I also found myself stopping CPR on someone I loved and sadly giving them up temporarily. As I looked up from the lifeless form of my twin brother, David, I thought, *I know where you'll be...I just better make sure I'm there as well.*

I think the same thing now about little Kaleb. I already can't wait to see him again, maybe even by my brother David's side, when things are finally finished down here.

Back home, I sob like a baby. Sarah walks in and kneels down in front of me. We embrace and cry together. Outside, the wind is blowing, whipping up a storm. It starts to rain.

God is crying too.

10 June 2009 PM
Coffin

When I first see the coffin it is half-finished. Lying amidst a pile of saw dust, it is a crude little thing, but somehow appropriate. Hard, twisted African mahogany has somehow been fashioned into a three foot long box. The bottom, back and sides seem to be waiting expectantly for the front and top in order to enclose a little boy's body.

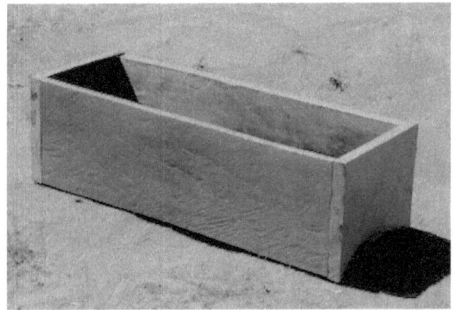

The Coffin

As I walk up to the container where Jeremy and Jonathan are making the coffin, I am struck by the cold beauty of the surroundings. A steel blue sky with gray angry clouds releases a slight drizzle of rain onto the African plain watering the wet sand and scrub bushes. A smattering of mango and Shea butter trees break up the monotony of the flat expanse. A group of tired grave diggers rest against the trunk of a tree to the right. Straight ahead is the beginnings of Gary's airplane hangar with the two old 20 foot containers making up the end of the hangar. Around the half-open doors of one container is gathered a crowd of mostly children with a smattering of adults all peering intently at the two white men making a coffin.

The purr of a small Honda generator is broken intermittently by the harsh roar of a power saw and the shocking pounding of large nails into hard wood. A cool breeze tries to soften the atmosphere which is heavy with grief.

I squeeze through the crowd just in time to help Jeremy and Jonathan lift up the coffin, measure around and make the final trimmings. The wood is so hard that holes have to be drilled before nailing or the nails will bend. We place the small head piece on and Jeremy hammers the nails home. The only thing left is to place a small boy, recently alive and well, into the interior and hammer the coffin shut until resurrection day.

The Adventist Youth Society has arrived in their sharp olive and tan uniforms. Jeremy, Jonathan and a couple of local men pick up the heavy burial box and lug it over to Gary and Wendy's humble abode. They place the casket gently on a simple wooden bed on the porch and wait for the final step.

Cherise, Gary and Wendy's two-and-a-half-year old daughter, runs in with a smile proudly showing off the cartoonish horse and car that Sarah has drawn on the back of her hands with a green marker.

It's almost time. Neighbors and friends are gathering outside. The rain continues to sprinkle the event as lighting flashes occasionally in the background. Gary looks at me. We walk silently over to the coffin and pick it up. It's rough and twisted wood bites into my hands with the weight of it's import crushing me more than it's physical gravitational force.

Followed by Wendy and Cherise we enter the house, pass through the living room and into the bedroom to the left where Kaleb awaits, cold and silent. He is peacefully lying on the floor next to the two mosquito net covered mattresses where he slept with his sister. A small, baby blanket covers most of his lifeless form.

Gary and I gently set the coffin down next to him. Gary lifts him up while Wendy arranges the blanket and smoothes it out over his face. Gary picks him up gently in his arms, tears streaming from his red and swollen eyes.

"Let me hold him one more time," Wendy's voice is deep and broken as she hugs her first born son for the last time on this earth.

"Cherise, do you want to kiss Kaleb one more time?" Gary asks softly.

"Yeah, daddy..." She approaches wiping away a stray strand of pure, blond hair from her cherubic face. She leans forward, lips puckered, and places a tiny kiss on the top of Kaleb's pale head.

Gary covers Kaleb up again and lays him in the coffin. He fits too well. This shouldn't be happening. I sob quietly, letting the tears flow freely.

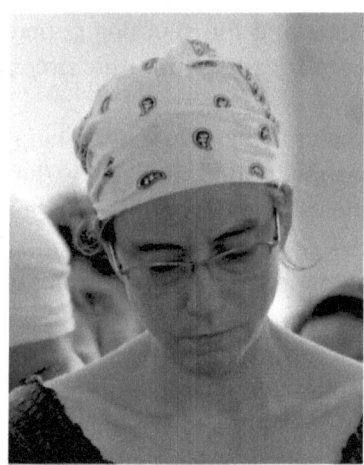

Wendy

We take the even heavier coffin out to the porch where Jeremy expertly pounds the last nails home with a devastating sound of finality. It's definitely time now.

The uniformed young people wait outside. Gary and I place the coffin on the shoulders of six young Tchadian girls who will bear the honors.

"*Gauche, gauche, gauche-droit-gauch...*" The solemn march begins as we all fall in behind the youth. They sing a mournful marching song about following Jesus no matter the cost. The words echo in the emptiness of the bush. The procession winds out the gate, around the fence, past the water tower and out towards the airstrip.

Gary's plane stares silently. Its windows are covered with a tarp. It's as if even it is too grief-stricken to observe the final steps of the young boy it knew so well. That boy will never again greet his daddy's return from mission flights or climb all over the cockpit dreaming of the day when he too will fly.

We march across the deep red laterite surface of the airstrip, cross a sandy path, pass through some low scrub brush and arrive at the six foot deep hole. This will be Kaleb's resting site until the end of the world. A pile of sandy clay with two hand made ropes strung across it lays to the side of the grave. The coffin is marched around the hole and deposited carefully on top of the ropes and dirt pile. A crowd has gathered. The wind blows. The rain falls. The universe mourns.

The service starts with a couple of French hymns that have never had much meaning for me until now:

> *Jusqu'à la mort, c'est notre cri de guerre,*
> *Le libre cri d'un peuple racheté,*
> *Jusqu'à la mort nous te serons fidèles.*

Even sung off tune, the deep feeling of those singing it penetrates to the bottom of my heart. *We are free. We are at war. There are casualties. But we don't mourn as those who have no hope. We will stay faithful.* My heart wants to believe it.

> *Et mon coeur n'a rien à craindre,*
> *Puisque tu me conduiras.*
> *Je te suivrai sans me plaindre*
> *En m'appuyant sur ton bras.*

A cold chill runs down my spine as I feel the presence of God. He is present. He weeps with us at this tragedy. We have nothing to fear.

I give opening prayer. André exhorts us with a little eulogy:

"Death is a sleep," he reminds us. "Our hope is in the resurrection when Jesus comes again to reunite all of us who have abandoned our rebellion against him. Kaleb's suffering is over. It's those of us left on earth who suffer. But Jesus is coming soon to wipe every tear from our eyes and destroy our last enemy...death."

Then, Gary talks about how much Kaleb loved to talk about Jesus and his second coming. Then he has us sing together Kaleb's favorite song in English:

> When the trumpet of the Lord shall sound,
> And time shall be no more...
> When the roll is called up yonder,
> I'll be there!

Unfortunately, as the local gravediggers go to lay the coffin in the tomb, they realize they've made the hole too small. They rush to and fro quickly to dig the grave larger. The chorale saves the day with a some traditional echo and repeat style African songs. Finally, the modifications are made. The coffin is slowly lowered into it's final resting place with the help of the rough ropes.

As the dirt starts to be shoveled on top of the coffin, Cherise seems to finally realize what's going on. Her heart-breaking cries and tears tear us all apart. Gary crouches down gently beside her.

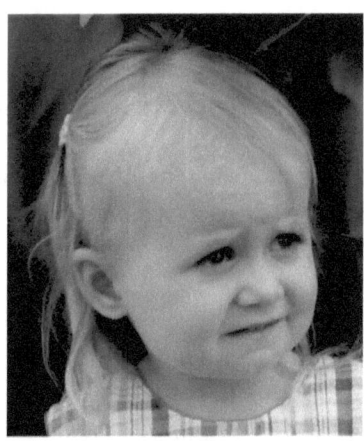

Cherise

"What is Kaleb doing right now?" Gary asks her.

"Sleeping, daddy."

"And when will he wake up?"

"Oh yeah, when Jesus comes." Her face lights up a little. She wipes her eyes as Wendy picks her up and holds her close.

As the crowd starts spontaneously singing in Nangjéré, the grave-diggers expertly create the funeral mound. A handmade hoe, a stick and the end of a shovel pound and stir the earth into place. Two other men shovel the earth in and continually pick up what has fallen to the sides. Some final pounding with the flats of the shovels creates a perfectly oval mound. Only those who've seen much death and assisted many funerals could make it so neatly.

We then turn to follow the Advent Youth as they lead us back singing the same marching songs. Arriving at the house, we follow local custom by seating Gary, Wendy and Cherise in lounge chairs. The other participants in the memorial service sit beside them while the mourners pass one by one to greet and offer their condolences.

The women curtsy and bow while solemnly shaking hands. As a sign of respect, they use both hands or the second hand touching the forearm of the right hand as they shake. The men shuffle and nod somberly as they hold Gary and Wendy's hands for a long time. They silently let you know they feel your loss, and they all have lost children so it means something. A crippled man on crutches hobbles in and hugs both parents while tears stream down his cheeks.

Finally, the kids file in for their respectful shaking of hands. The adults take a seat on mats spread out behind the choral which has been singing French hymns without ceasing. Annie and some of the local women serve Kool-Aid. People quietly converse. Occasional sobs burst forth. Laughter is sometimes heard. Gary and Wendy are periodically called away by phone calls from well-wishers around the world.

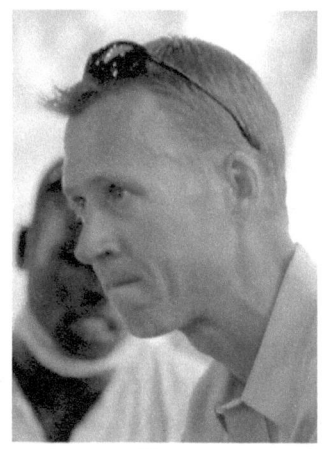

Gary

Dusk approaches. Noel rises and calls an end to the wake with a prayer. The locals graciously don't insist on their custom of singing, dancing and drumming all night long. Instead, everyone files solemnly out shaking our hands one last time. About this time, Rich and Anne, our friends from N'Djamena arrive.

Finally, the sun sets on a day that should never have been. It started out as any other day. Then it quickly degenerated into an early morning ER call, a desperate last ditch effort and the laying to rest of a four year old boy in a crude, twisted coffin. Now he will rest peacefully in the African bush through what's left of this world's turmoil. He will sleep until the end of the world and the beginning of the next.

Then God will wipe away every tear from our eyes...

23 June 2009
Only God Knows

I've just started rounds on surgery. The young girl operated on for perforated bowel secondary to Typhoid Fever is doing much better. She still has a drain in. We're doing dressing changes on the infected skin incision. But she's eating, drinking, walking, pooping and peeing.

Suddenly, Carson comes to see me.

"We need ya' to help us fin' an IV on a kid...it's kinda urgent," he tells me in his slow drawl.

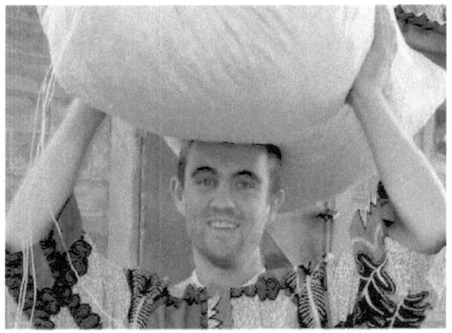

Carson (aka Mel Gibson)

I walk through the open screen door, across the porch covered with convalescing patients lying on colorful mats, through the well-swept courtyard and over to the sidewalk.

A small crowd has gathered around a mother with a brightly colored head wrap holding a limp child. They sit on a wooden chair facing away from me. A white coated nurse bends closely over the child trying to start an IV. It's Tchibtchang. Standing to the side, muscles bulging out of his scrubs, Abel holds a bottle of 5% glucose attached to an IV line waiting for the chance to attach it to venous access.

Carson fills me in as we walk up. "Really low blood sugar. Sick for a week. Treated at home with market meds and who knows what else. Just came in. Unconscious. We can't get an IV."

The kid's eyes are rolled back in his head. His hands and face are pale. His body is like a rag doll. I listen and he has a faint heart beat. He's barely breathing.

"Abel, let's get him to the operating room!"

Abel grabs the child. We rush off around the corner and into the brightly lit prep room. Abel places the child on a gurney and I start doing chest compressions. Abel and Tchibtchang try to find a scalp vein. Carson is holding the bottle of IV fluids. I've started a subcutaneous infusion on his abdomen which is swelling up. He remains unconscious.

"Try the external jugular vein on his neck," I suggest to Abel and Tchibtchang.

Augustin arrives and tries as well. No success. I try a femoral vein on both sides while Abel and Carson take turns doing CPR. I fail on both sides.

The nurses keep trying on the scalp and neck. No luck. I call for another hemoglobin. I can't believe the first one is really 10.0 g/dl. He looks too pale. His heart is still beating, though barely. We keep up CPR.

The boy is about two and a half years old. His mom stands in the background, a helpless and hopeless expression on her face. She's probably thinking of all the other small boys she's seen buried in her life. I'm thinking about the little boy I just buried a couple weeks ago. I look at the mom and our eyes meet.

I'm about ready to stop. *This never works anyway*. The hemoglobin comes back 8.0 g/dl. We keep on doing CPR. The nurses keep trying to find an IV. I finally try the right femoral vein again.

I stretch out the skin on his inner thigh. I feel for a pulse but find nothing. I poke blindly with a 22G IV catheter attached to a syringe I aspirate from. I get some dark blood back. I can't really thread the catheter. I take out the needle. No blood. I slowly pull it back until the blood starts to ooze out.

"Bring me the glucose!" I call.

Carson hands me the IV tubing. He holds it while the solution runs in fast. Abel tapes it down but has to hold it in a certain position or it doesn't work. Within 30 seconds, the boy's eyes open. A few seconds later he's looking around and starting to move his limbs. He has a strong heart beat and is breathing!

We give him some sugar water orally. Tchibtchang explains to the mom that she needs to make sure he drinks the sweet solution all day long. We let the IV glucose run in. Augustin finally finds a real IV. I have them start a Quinine drip for malaria.

Why do some make it and some don't? God only knows.

27 June 2009

Horses

It's a gray Saturday morning and a cool breeze is blowing . A cloudy sky brings out the deepness of the green starting to push up through the desert soil. The transformation of desert into lush grasslands has begun with the first rains.

Stefan and I are going for a ride. Pepper and Bob are standing near the stables, but Libby is nowhere to be found. I search the compound and finally find her standing under a tree staring blankly through the chain link fence across the soccer field into the horizon. I grab her halter. She resists briefly with her head pulled back before resigning herself to her fate.

I tie Bob up to the tree right outside the stables and grab the new, synthetic saddle someone just gave Sarah. I cinch it up as tight as I can across Bob's ever increasing girth. He's getting so strong I'll use the bit today. I first place the bit into his mouth. Then I slide the rest of the beautifully worked leather and silver harness over his ears and attach it under his chin. I throw the saddle bag over Libby's rump and fill it with water bottles, a French Bible and a Nangjéré songbook. I place my left foot into Bob's stirrup and swing up into the saddle.

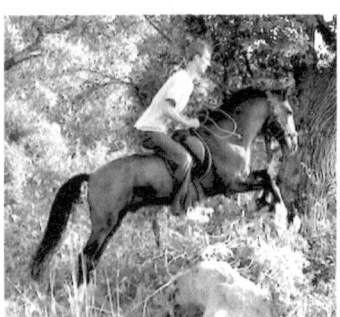

James & Bob

Stefan and I saunter up to the gate and out into the street. Most people are just waking up. They huddle around smoky leaf fires warming themselves up after a long, cold night. Some are gathered around a pot of *bouillie*. They anticipate a temporary assuaging of the ever present hunger at the end of the dry season.

We cross Béré and approach Bendélé. Gary and Wendy's empty house stares at us from the left. Its gate is locked with a padlock. Its windows are barred. A heavy silence reigns.

A hundred meters further on, Noel's children wave and flash huge grins as they shout out *"Lapia! James-uh! Stef-ahn!"*

Passing Noel's house takes us out of the village and into the bush. The main road is packed with a steady procession of people on their way to the market. Women in brightly colored wraps saunter along. Their arms swing in rhythm keeping the large basins filled with sweet potatoes, sugar, millet, rice, corn, bean leaves and other marketable items balanced on their heads.

An ox cart plods slowly by loaded with sacks of grain. A few young kids are piled on top and one lazily sits across the pulling bar with a stick in hand. From time to time, he swats the two long-horned cows in the right direction.

More women pass, long piles of twisted sticks cut into six feet lengths, tied and bundled onto their heads. Old and young mix in a never ending procession heading for the biggest event of the week, the Béré market.

Soon, we enter a small village. Some of the travelers have stopped under a mango tree and are gathered around a large pot of freshly prepared rice wine. They fill their bellies for the exhausting trip to Béré on foot. The alcohol also prepares themselves for the social scene. Eventually, they will stagger home, dead drunk. They wave to us wildly Their faces light up with white, toothy grins as we pass and call out our greetings.

Stefan and I stop to switch horses. He was having some troubles controlling Libby. We start trotting when a stretch of road opens up before us. I give a cluck and a kick with my heels. Libby responds and we are off at a fast gallop. She's the newest addition to our stables. Like Pepper and Bob, she came at a good price, thanks to her malnourishment. When Sarah walked her back from the Arab village where we bought her, she could barely do the five kilometers at a slow walk. She's put on some weight and become one of the friendliest horses around. Now, I want to see if she can run and if she's competitive.

I'm in front for a while before Bob catches up and passes us. Libby picks up speed a little, but seems to have no urge to pass Bob. Alternately walking, trotting and galloping the 18 kilometers to Delbian pass quickly. We are bombarded along the way with a thousand *"Lapias"* and *"As-salaamu aleikums"*.

Stefan and I tie up Libby and Bob near some grass. A short man with a limp brings a bucket, fills it at the local water pump and gives the horses a much needed drink. We take off the saddles and hang them over mango tree branches out of the reach of curious little hands.

I get to tell the story of David and Goliath to a group of kids who gather about. Practically every other boy is carrying his own sling and sheep are grazing in the background. The story of a shepherd boy killing a giant with a stone and sling has never seemed more real.

Noel tells me that I'll be preaching to the group of adults that's gathered for worship. I borrow a sermon I heard on tape from a missionary in New Guinea. I talk about God loving impossibilities. He used Gideon and 300 men to fight off an army of 135,000. He motivated Elijah to challenge 400 prophets of Baal on a mountain to a duel. Finally, God saved Daniel's three friends from a fiery furnace when they stood up against the king of Babylon and his entire staff.

In a surprising lack of African hospitality, Stefan and I are allowed to skip lunch. For us, it's an escape from the usual obligatory millet paste and slimy fish sauce meal. So we head back to Béré. Just outside of Dabegue, we come across three young boys riding bareback on tiny ponies herding cattle.

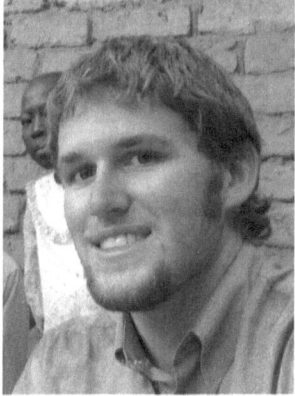

Stefan

As we trot past, one of them turns and starts running alongside heading towards the road. He wants to race! I cluck loudly and give a big kick to Libby's flanks. She almost shoots out from under me as she pushes to catch the pony. Within seconds we pull even and leave the surprisingly fast pony in the dust.

Entering Dabegue we tear around puddles of water, under trees and around people scampering to get out of the way. I'd seen Stefan gunning Bob and was sure he'd catch us by now. I look quickly over my shoulder and he's nowhere to be found. Giving a commanding "whoa" I pull back sharply on the reins and lean back with all my force. Libby stops dead in her tracks.

Stefan finally catches up. "I lost my hat when Bob took off," he explains. We continue trotting and walking until we are about five kilometers from Béré.

"Let's race Bob and Libby," I say. "I want to really see what she can do. See that tree to the left just beyond that puddle? It'll be a walk up start. As soon as we enter the shadow of the tree, the race starts."

I feel my heart beat pick up as the tree approaches. We try to keep the horses even. It's a slow walk up. We're only a few feet away. The horses start to sense our excitement...and...we're there.

Libby seems to have been expecting it. She rockets forward almost pulling my feet out of the stirrups. I'm holding on for dear life. We're ahead! I see Bob out of the corner of my eye cut to the left where a side path goes around some bushes. He's picking up speed. At the same time I feel Libby fading, she's just not in shape and running out of energy. Bob leaves us way behind. Libby and I continue a slow gallop to the entrance to the town of Béré. I pull her up and we do a cool-down walk the rest of the way home.

When I finally pull myself out of the saddle, I can't believe how tired I am. I'm so wobbly I can barely stand. I'm covered with sweat and fine dust. The horses slurp up bucketfuls of water and then go for a roll as soon as their saddles are off. I take a quick shower and fall into a deep sleep.

I'm soon wakened by Hortence at the door. "There's a woman with high blood pressure and seizures. She's seven months pregnant. The cervix is completely dilated."

I give some instructions and go back down to lie down. I soon think better of it, get up, put on scrubs and head to the hospital.

In the labor and delivery room the woman is thrashing around on the bed moaning and whining. The cervix is only at three centimeters. We start an oxytocin drip to give her better contractions. I go to see some other patients. Hortence comes running to get me.

"She's having a crisis again!"

I go back to labor and delivery. The woman's husband is at her side. The woman is hysterical. It's not a seizure, though, and she quickly calms down when the husband leaves. I order some pain medication and then she has a full seizure in my presence. Hortence and I wheel her in the gurney to the operating room.

Fortunately, Siméon is already at the hospital. Samedi lives right next door. David runs to get them. The woman is combative and agitated and difficult to get on the operating room table. We tie her arms and legs down good. While Siméon preps the abdomen, Samedi and I scrub.

Samedi prays. Siméon gives one milliliter of Ketamine, I slice down to fascia, rip the fascia and muscles open, lift up a bladder flap, slice into the uterus, poke into the amniotic sac and squeeze out a full term baby boy After a little rubbing and slapping, he gives a healthy cry. I suture up the uterus and skin and head home to finally rest.

30 June 2009
Snakebite

The sound of a loud diesel motor and the sudden appearance of headlights outside shocks me out of a deep sleep. I awaken to the darkness of a moonless Tchadian night. The truck stops in front of the hospital. I have a feeling I might as well get up already.

Sure enough, within minutes, the all-too-familiar *knock, knock, knock* on the sheet metal door confirms my suspicions.

"*Oui*?" I mumble as I roll out of bed trying not to disturb Sarah.

"*C'est moi!*" Sounds out from through the screen door, across the porch and into the bedroom. It sounds like Augustin. I pull on some shorts, grab my glasses and fumble through the semi-darkness. Fortunately, the living room is lit by the eery blue light of a bug lamp.

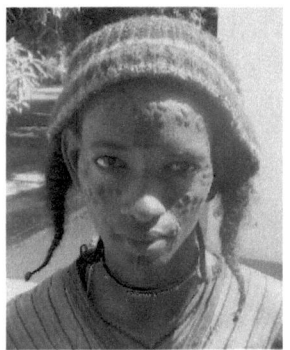

Fulani boy

"They've just brought in a Fulani boy with a snake bite."

I arrive at the door and take the blue *carnet* from Augustin's outstretched arm.

"He's agitated and his leg is swollen," he adds.

"How long has it been?" I ask.

"About two hours. They're camped out over by Lai. He went to get some water or something and was bit on the foot."

"How did they find a car at this hour?" I wonder aloud, rubbing my eyes sleepily.

"One of them ran to Lai and found someone," explains Augustin.

"Ok, give him a vial of anti-venom in 500mL of Ringer's. Let it run in over 30 minutes. There's not much else really to do. Either it'll work or it won't...oh, and give him some Diazepam to calm him down."

"*C'est bon,*" agrees Augustin and disappears into the night.

I walk inside and pour some water into a canning jar. The jar serves as my guide to make sure I drink at least five liters of water a day. As I stare out into the shadows of the yard my thoughts wander to the boy bit by the snake.

Should I go up to the hospital? Would it make a difference? Won't he just probably die anyway?

I start to think of the two forces in this world, good and evil. *Which would want me to go up to the hospital? And which would recommend I go back to sleep? Put that way, it's a no-brainer...* I put on scrubs, grab my keys and head up to the ER.

On the way I send up a quick prayer. *Whatever happens, make sure You get the glory. If I can pray with them, give me the chance so they'll recognize You as the One who heals.*

I arrive in the ER and pull back the green and yellow curtain. Writhing on the bed in agony—looking like death warmed over—is a slender, wiry nomad boy. He has dreads, traditional scarring on his face, leather fetish bags around his neck, string bracelets on his wrists and wild colored pants with blood staining the right leg. His right ankle is covered with blood-soaked gauze and the entire leg is swollen and already blistering.

He is moaning and non-responsive. His gums are bleeding. From time to time he thrashes around.

A shaven headed man in a dark gray pant-suit, traditional tattoos and the obligatory leather pouches around the neck comes up. What is remarkable is that he doesn't have dreads. On top of that, he has a cell phone sticking out of his shirt pocket safely secured with a string around his neck. He stands at the head of the bed.

Squatting all around the ER are more Fulani men and several women. All of them have the crazy dreads and black, charcoal based lined tattoos on the face, arms and chest. Plastic shoes are standard. Another family member stands in a corner, the bottom of his left foot pushed against his inner right thigh as he balances on one foot like a flamingo.

Augustin arrives with the IV. I hold the boy's left arm still while he gets the IV perfusion running.

"Give him an ampoule of Pentazocine sub-cue," I add. "Since obviously the Diazepam isn't enough."

As Augustin leaves to get the Pentazocine I motion to the Fulani men and speak to them in my broken Arabic.

"We pray to Allah," I motion with my hands outstretched, palms up. "Allah give him health. *Allah wahid*, ok?"

Heads nod vigorously in agreement as arms outstretch in the Muslim prayer position.

"*Rabbina Allah!* Give this boy health. Give this boy life. In the name of *Isa al-Masih, Amin!*"

As the simple prayer finishes our hands move to our faces to take in Allah's blessing. "*Shukran,*" "*Inshallah*" and "*Al hamdullilah*" reverberate around the sleeping, snake-bit boy. The bald man points to the sky and pronounces solemnly, "Allah only gives health and life. *Allah wahid.*"

Augustin arrives and gives the Pentazocine. I go to the operating room and get a 60mL syringe. Back in the ER, I draw up 20mL of Ringers and combine it with the 10mL of anti-venom. I give it slow IV push over ten minutes. Within minutes of starting the anti-venom, the gingival bleeding stops and the ankle bleeding slows down.

The boy is asleep now, thanks to the meds. In fact, he's gurgling. I show the Fulani man with the bald head how to do a jaw thrust to open his airway and the boy starts breathing easier. I keep reminding him to keep the airway open as he keeps getting distracted. Finally, he buckles down and gets it right.

I tell Augustin to get some IV Chlorpheniramine ready in case he has an allergic reaction. He comes back to say that the pharmacy is out.

Just then, I notice some welts showing up on the boys arms and abdomen. I rush to the operating room and come back with Adrenaline and Benadryl. Augustin gives him the shots. The rash stops spreading. The boy's heart is racing and he's still unconscious.

I go back to the operating room into the stock room. After searching a bit I find the Hydrocortisone I'm looking for. We just bought it last week at the pharmacy in Lai. Augustin adds 100mg to the perfusion.

I stay by the boy's side. I periodically place my hand on his chest to feel his heart beat and see if he has a fever. He's breathing is slow and shallow. Without the constant pressure of his Fulani uncle's hands thrusting his lower jaw forward, he would drown in his own saliva.

What I wouldn't give for an old foot powered suction pump!

The bleeding has all but stopped. The hives aren't spreading and they even seem to be receding a little. The Fulani faces around me seem to relax a little. They sense that he might live.

"*Al hamdullilah!*" I say and point skyward. "*Allah!*"

I go home.

The next morning, the boy starts to wake up. We find he also has malaria. After three more days of malaria treatment, he is eating, sitting up, moving around and the swelling in his leg has started to go down.

As I bid them farewell on the day of his discharge I shout after them, "*Al hamdulillah! Allah al-Kerim!*"

26 July 2009
Inshallah

I'm in an SUV with a group of Muslims roaring across the desert towards Eastern Tchad. Our destination is Abéché, the center for the humanitarian efforts for the Sudanese refugees from Darfur.

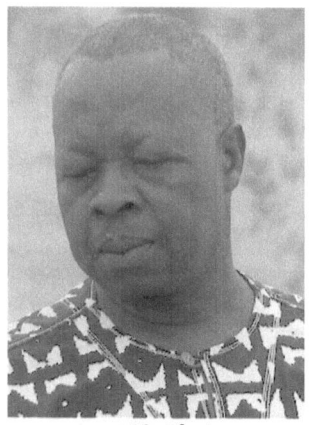

Aimé

Aimé's colleague, Mahamat Saleh Abakar, has invited me to come see his village. Both Aimé and Mahamat Saleh are constitutional advisors to the President of Tchad. Mahamat Saleh told Aimé he'd heard what the

Adventists are doing in Béré and wondered if we couldn't come out to Eastern Tchad. I've always wanted to see that part of the country, so I readily agree. Deep down, though, I have no interest in another project. Between Béré and Moundou, I've got my hands full.

We pass Bedouin caravans heading north. Women in brightly colored body wraps and head scarves boast huge gold nose rings. They frantically beat their donkeys to get them to move off the road as we come cruising past. Robed, turbaned and bearded men lumber by swaying on the backs of heavily loaded camels, bounce along on horseback or plod along on foot chasing the goats and sheep. Most are armed with bows and arrows, spears or staffs. Tucked away in their robes one is sure to find the ever present dagger. Many probably have rifles hidden in their saddle bags.

Dried up animals in various states of decomposition litter the shoulders of the highway. Poor rainfall this year has led to famine and the loss of cattle, donkeys, horses and other vital livestock. Occasionally the smell of a rotting carcass sneaks it's way in through the windows of our passing vehicles.

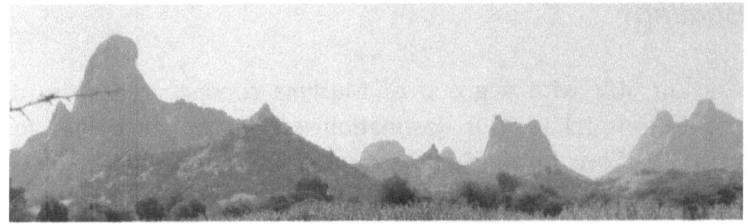

The road to Abéché

The African plain starts to be interrupted by wadis, rolling hills and piles of boulders. In the distance, jagged peaks and granite outcroppings break up the horizon. We enter the central Tchadian Sahel where rain has been more abundant and the grasslands are bright green. Crops of millet are starting to push their way out of the soil. Local farmers dig up the ground with small spades on the end of long poles. Women coming back from the fields carry water and rations in woven net bags suspended from poles slung across one shoulder. No one carries things balanced on top of their heads like they do in Béré and the rest of the South.

We stop by the side of the road for a picnic. One of the drivers pours us tea and sweetened milk from thermoses as we wait in the shade of a thorny desert scrub tree. A platter of grilled chicken and French baguettes is shared among our two groups of five.

We continue on with regular stops for tea, milk and ritual prayer. One stop for prayer finds us in the midst of a cluster of mountains and date palms. The prayer rugs are rolled out and the absolution's begun in front of a man slicing up a sheep into large portions to be roasted on a piece of tin roofing suspended over a wood fire.

We spend the night in Mongo at the World Food Program compound and are up before five for morning prayers, milk, tea and Tchadian beignets. We arrive late in the afternoon at Abeche, Tchad's fourth largest city.

As we enter the mud brick compound and seat ourselves on enormous mats, I experience for the first time what an Arabic greeting really is. A rhythmic, staccato exchange of words proceeds for at least five minutes repeating *mashallah* at least 20 times and *Al hamdullilah* at least 15 times. For variety and flavor, one can throw in countless other words asking about health for everybody, strength, improvement, etc.

I soon join in and find it very satisfying. Hands are shook during most of the greeting, eyes look down and occasionally the hand is released to bring one's own hand in to touch the chest over the heart before reaching out again to take the other's hand in greeting. To end the salutation, one releases the hand and slowly sits down on the mat letting one's *mashallah* and *al hamdullilah* slowly fade out.

Adding to the milk and tea we now have Arabic coffee, *qahweh,* seasoned with cardamom. We also have *boule* to eat with some of the best sauces I've had in Tchad: ground meat with lots of cumin and okra.

I take a shower in a walled in corner next to a poop hole. I step up on a small raised platform and pour water on myself from a bucket. Just outside, in the other corner, about 20 small girls are learning to recite the Qur'an. Their sweet voices blend together in a cacophony of different rhythms as none of them is in sync with the other. It is beautiful and cute. It feels good to splash water on myself and wash the red dust off my face, arms and hair.

The men stretch out and sleep together on the mats in the men's courtyard where the women don't dare to enter. Whenever a female family member has arrived she starts her greeting standing. Then she kneels down just outside the low wall of the courtyard. The male family member goes outside to greet her and kneels down beside her for the prolonged ritual greeting.

The morning starts with prayer at sunrise, approximately 4:30am. I read some passages of scripture while my Muslim friends do the *salat.* Then we drink milk, eat beignets and head out to see the local authorities.

First stop is the governor. Mahamat Saleh, explains that he's invited us out to look at the possibility of opening a medical center in his village. The

Governor doesn't seem to keen since there's a health center in the neighboring town of Abougoudam.

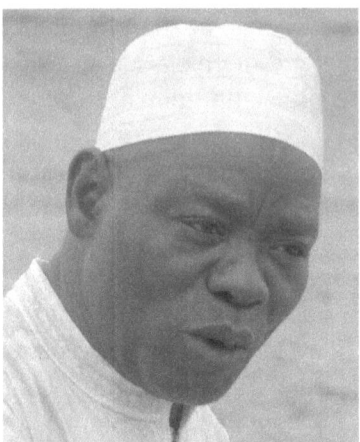

Mahamat Saleh Abakar

However, when Mahamat Saleh explains that it will be more than a health center, more like a hospital, the Governor reluctantly gives his ok. On walking out with his *Directeur du Cabinet*, we receive a much warmer reception. The lighter skinned man with obvious Arabic features dressed in an ample robe and white turban beams a smile.

"I'm from the same village," he says. "I'll do everything I can to help you get the paperwork pushed through for the land and anything else you need."

The Prefect and Sultan are out of town so we head out of Abeche towards Abougoudam. There we plan to see the Sous-prefect, the chief political figure of the group of villages surrounding Abougoudam .

The Sous-prefect welcomes us into his old, colonial-style, thick-walled mansion. Unfortunately, it looks like it hasn't been maintained since independence in 1960. We sit down on mats, eat goat meat and drink tea, *qahweh,* and Coke. Directly in front of us is a room stacked to the ceiling with cement, all that's left of a project to build the sous-prefect a new house. Apparently, the rest of the supplies where stolen by bandits who assassinated the builder.

We follow the sous-prefect out to the village where he shows us a flat, barren stretch of ground he wants to give us. It doesn't feel right. We move on to where Mahamat Saleh and his brother, Mahamat Hassan, have drilled a well for their village. Next to the pump are three dried out cattle carcasses. The water came a little too late for them. About ten boys mounted bareback on horses have come to water their flocks.

I point to a fairly close plateau next to a small mountain: "That's more what I'm interested in."

"That's in another county," says Mahamat Saleh. We have no influence there...it won't work."

We seem at an impasse when a local man almost hidden by his enormous turban rattles off something quickly in Arabic. We hop back in the SUVs and head a little out of Mahamat Saleh's village towards another village. The village is called Argoudi. There we find a small hill crowned with huge boulders that is not in use. In all directions stretches the African plain broken up by wadis and scrub brush. The mountains in the distance ring us in on all sides. It's perfect. They are happy and agree to give us ten hectares.

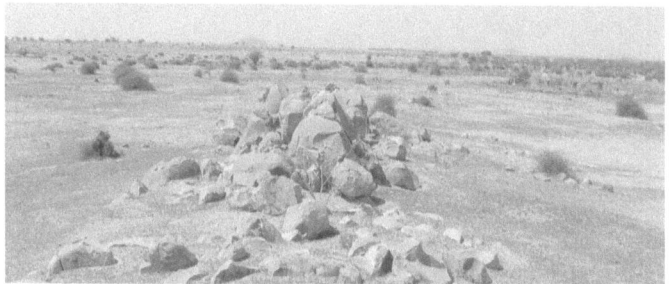

Site of future Adventist Hospital near Abéché

That evening, I speak with Yacoub Abdoulaye, Mahamat Saleh's cousin.

"What's the hospital in Abeche like?" I ask. "For example, how's the surgery service?"

"Well, let's put it this way," says Yacoub. "If ten people are operated on, five will live, five will die. Plus, often people die in the hallways of the hospital without even being seen by a doctor or nurse because they have no money."

That coincides with what I'd heard last week in N'Djamena from a German midwife working at an orphanage in Abeche.

"A few weeks ago," she said. "During a single week, three women died during c-sections. Most of our orphans are orphans because of their mothers dying in childbirth. It's not AIDS or the refugee crisis or the war...it's almost complete lack of obstetrical care during deliveries."

Back in Mahamat Saleh's courtyard, an old Arab man with a skull cap, white robe and a wizened face with years of smile wrinkles speaks up.

"Daktor, shifah al kat-kat da," he says as he shows me his lab slip and prescription.

He has malaria and a negative Typhoid test and wants me to explain. He was prescribed Typhoid fever treatment anyway along with five other meds including quinine for malaria. The total was the equivalent of $50, a quarter of a month's wages. To top it off, the pharmacy hadn't filled the prescription right. Instead of the prescribed Quinine, he was actually given Chloroquine, which is no longer an effective treatment for malaria.

That night, a funeral next door allows all the local young Imams in training to practice their oral recitation of the Qur'an...with a microphone and speakers. It goes on all night long until 6:00am the next morning. I am alternately soothed by those who have the talent and annoyed by those who seem to be screeching like dying mules trying to sing the otherwise beautiful Arabic of the Qur'an. But, I sleep well anyway.

On the way back, Mahamat Saleh tells us a story:

A man gets up one morning to go to the market. He fishes his money out from under the mattress and sticks it in his pocket.

"I'm going to the market to buy a donkey," he says to his wife.

"Inshallah," she responds.

Halfway out the door, the man looks back at her. "Inshallah? If God wills it? What has God got to do with it? I've got money in my pocket and there are plenty of donkeys at the market. I'm going to buy one. Keep your inshallah to yourself."

With that he slams the door and marches off. Halfway to the market, he is waylaid by bandits who tie him up and take his money. They leave him under a tree all day. When it's dark, the man manages to free himself. He makes his way slowly back to his house where he finds the door locked. He knocks on the door.

"Who's there?" His wife asks from inside.

"Open the door, it's me your husband...inshallah!"

Two days of traveling later, I finally pull up to the Béré Adventist Hospital. For some reason, I'm reminded of the story. I pray silently that the doors will continue to open for us to have a hospital there in Eastern Tchad...*inshallah*!

09 August 2009
Moonlight

As I stare out into the moonlight filtering through the flamboyant tree branches casting shifting shadows with every breath of wind...

As I hear the soft shuffle and breathing of our sweat-flecked horses outside the stable...

As I draw my gaze back to the pile of pineapple carvings in front of the cutting board and bring the ice-cold pineapple to my mouth, slowly savoring crunching into the juicy morsel...

As I think back over the past few days I find it incredible to think of how this afternoon ended...

I can only call it an unexpected grace, a surprising joy, a metaphysical moment when all things good come together out of the midst of all things wrong...

I'm galloping through the forest, grasping Pepper's mane as fiercely as I hold to the reins. I stand up in the stirrups and hug my body to the horse's powerful neck. Leaves slap my face. A branch rips through the skin of my shoulder. The full moon lights up the sandy trail like a river of silver stretching lazily out before me through the dark shadows of the trees. My sweat soaked shirt clings to my back. I am surrounded by the silence of an African evening in the bush. I'm carried away beyond the horrors, sorrows and sufferings of the last few days...

I notice the remarkably strong features of the handsome Arab man. He stares steadfastly upward with a look of incomprehensible peace. A dozen turbaned comrades lug him up the ramp to the operating room. He lies in a vinyl stretcher with wooden handles held firmly in the grips of his friends. His mangled body is wrapped in a blood soaked turban, a stark contrast to the serenity of his gaze.

I spend hours working on his bilateral open fibula and tibia fractures. The bones on the right are laid bare by a flap of skin running from his heel up his calf and across the top of his foot. The anatomy couldn't be clearer: muscles, tendons, ligaments and bones. It brings back memories from Anatomy lab in medical school.

He calmly complains of neck pain. He can't move or feel his body from the neck down. It is a silent grace allowing us to work on his tattered limbs without anesthesia. I frame his chiseled face in a cervical collar and get to work.

I feel I'll never survive the emotional roller coaster of the myriads of visitors. The robed, turbaned men and brightly wrapped women in head scarves file incessantly in and out. Many of the men leave with tears unashamedly rolling down their cheeks. I try to console them.

"*Fi iden Allah*, leave it in God's hands," I say. "Only He knows the day of our death. Trust Him."

I have to fight my way through crowds and over colorful mats and rugs to get to him in the wards. I do his complicated dressings after spending what seems like ages of emotional energy trying to get the swarming family and friends to respect visiting hours and hospital policies.

After three days, his paralysis is unchanged. I'm almost relieved when Tchibtchang comes to get me in the morning.

"*Ça ne va pas.*"

I arrive at his bedside in time to see his unconscious, but still dignified face take it's last shallow breath. I feel his heart beat in his neck slow down and become weak. He was bound for a long road of suffering as a quadriplegic. It is certainly God's mercy that has laid him to sleep.

I stand on the bank of the river, looking down on the swirling eddies of the brown, engorged river. I see the sun slowly set behind the great branching trees of the African plain. I turn around and see the full moon rising through a circle made by two rounded trees and a small hill. I watch the slow transformation of the day into moonlit night. I feel the wet of the river slowly drying on my body. I watch Stefan desperately trying to capture the moment on film. Eddie slowly makes his way upstream against the current. I pull on my jeans over my moist swimming suit and prepare for the ride home. I untangle Pepper from the bush I've tied him to. I am amazed at how quickly depression and overwhelming burnout can be replaced by wonder, marvel and ecstasy.

Is it possible that only this morning I found myself deep in a belly under the ribs carefully cauterizing a gallstone filled gallbladder from the liver of an elderly Muslim man?

Is it possible that yesterday I was about to throw up but finally gave in and started taking malaria treatment only to go out immediately and take out an ovarian tumor stuck to all the intestines, omentum and uterus?

Is it possible that only two days ago I didn't think I'd make it through the morning much less the week because of fatigue I refused to believe was another bout of *Plasmodium falciparum* destroying my blood cells?

Is it possible that only three days ago the hospital was full to overflowing while we spent all of a Sunday afternoon filling it up with sick babies needing blood transfusions and malaria treatment?

Is it possible that only four days ago I spent all Saturday in the operating room with two motorcycle accidents needing emergent orthopedic intervention?

I come back from work and almost collapse. It's been another day of never-ending hospital rounds, complicated surgeries, ER patients, ultrasounds—all pleasantly muffled with the ringing of Quinine in my ears. I feel a little nauseated and drink some cold water. I sit down and finish reading *Flying Doctor of the Philippines*. I just want to sleep, but decide I better go out and feed the horses to keep my wife happy.

The next thing I know, I'm in the saddle trotting past the mud huts of Béré, around the pond, through the forest and onto the river road mounted on Pepper. Behind me, Stefan rides Bob and Eddie rides Libby. Out into the open Stefan and Eddie cluck their horses into a gallop. I can feel Pepper tensing beneath me. I release him with a yell and a squeeze of my thighs. He quickly closes the gap. We pass the others by going straight through a mud puddle while Bob goes left around it and Libby goes right.

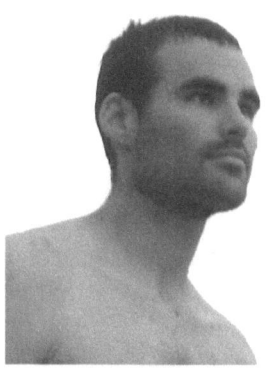

Eddie

We're in the open now and I slow down. I see the river. We ride down the ridges gauged out by the rain leading to the cattle crossing and then climb up the hill next to it. We dismount and tie up the horses.

A quick assessment confirms the possibilities. Eddie and I strip down. I look at the cliff then back at Eddie. I squint and we both race off the cliff. Arms and legs flailing wildly, I crash into the swift moving current below.

Eddie wants more. We pull our reluctant bodies up the bank using exposed tree roots.

We climb a tree as high as possible. There's still a path clear of branches to the rushing waters below. I crouch on two diverging limbs my hands in front. I propel myself through the gap, past the other branches below and into the welcoming arms of the cool, refreshing liquid beneath. As I surface, I remember why I'm glad there are no crocs and lions in this part of Africa.

After multiple jumps, Eddie and I climb up the bank for the last time. Stefan's face is glowing. It's hard to believe just last night he was talking about maybe wanting to leave. His joy is contagious.

"The only thing that could make this better," he says laughing. "Would be a little bit of ice cream."

Later, as I walk through the cool of the moonlit evening from my house to his carrying the plate of chilled fruit I think to myself, *Well, cold pineapple could arguably be as good or better...*

Back at my house, the clapping of hands comes again.

"There's an old man," says Salomon. "He's been peeing blood since this morning..."

I head back to the hospital. Moonlight leads the way.

14 August 2009
SIGN

It's 3:46am and I can't sleep. My eyes are bloodshot and heavy. My head pounds. But I can't sleep. Jet lag is at it again. I huddle under the blankets to keep from freezing in the air conditioned hotel room in Richland, Washington. It's hard to imagine that just a few sleepless days ago I was in the bush of the Sahel.

The trip consists of a simple six hour bus ride from Béré to N'Djamena, a five hour overnight flight to Paris, 45 minutes to Amsterdam and an eleven hour direct flight to Seattle. I meet Greg in the airport. We grab a rental car and drive over the mountains covered with pines and firs into the central valley. We pass through rolling golden hills, small farming towns and roadside stands selling fresh, cold cherries. Following a smaller river south, we eventually hit the Columbia River at the Tri Cities. Richland is one of the three cities. We've arrived for the SIGN Orthopedic conference.

I get out of bed at about 4:30am, strap on my running shoes and head out the door. The night is just beginning to turn a lighter shade of black. The well-lit streets need no natural light. I run across a road around a middle school. Sprinklers caress the school's well manicured lawns, soccer and football fields. Down a side street I head off road up a grassy slope and onto the riverside walking trail.

The scent of sage, mountain misery, pine and fir wafts across the early morning breeze. If not for the vigorous sweat I've already worked up on my out of shape body, I'd probably be chilled to the bone. A grove of trees and dense shrubbery gives me only glimpses of the dark, alabaster surface of the river. I turn a corner and see an opening leading down a pebbly bank onto a small sandy beach. I stumble down and after some pushups squat on the sand to reflect.

Yesterday, on the first day of the conference, I found myself surrounded by an international aura of languages. Urdu, Hindi, Vietnamese, Slavic, Arabic, French, and Spanish swirled around me complemented by a wide variety of English accents from Nigeria, Cameroon, Tanzania, Kenya, India, Bangladesh, Mongolia, England and the United States.

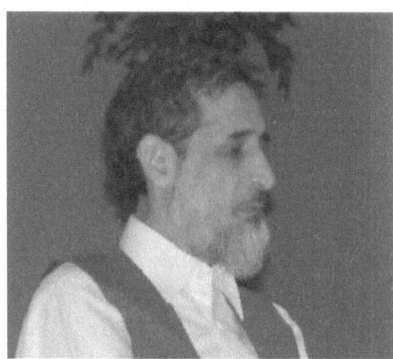

Dr. Shah

One of the presenters is the slender Dr. Shah from Pakistan. He has an ample gray beard and thin, fierce face with a long pointed nose. Starting during the terrible earthquake in northern Pakistan and continuing on today in some of the most remote areas of the world, Dr. Shah has done more than 1000 intramedullary SIGN nails for long bone fractures.

Another presenter, the dignified, dark skinned Dr. Faruque from Bangladesh speaks with a half smile calmly out from under his mop of black hair.

Dr. Shahab from Peshawar lectures us elegantly on bomb blast injuries. His portly figure fits well in his classy suit. A well-trimmed white beard frames his jolly face, outlining his dark features.

We go on a tour of the machine shop where intramedullary rods, screws and instruments are made at a fraction of the competitors' prices but with the same levels of quality control. I enter into a workshop where 20 artificial femurs and an equal number of tibias await our inexperienced hands.

An orthopedist from Vietnam leads a small group of conference attendees, including Greg and I, through the process of inserting a SIGN nail. He explains how to attach the target arm to the rod and adjust it so the distal fixating screws will be able to be placed without intra-operative imagery. He demonstrates how to insert the nail into the bone with frequent side to side sweeps interspersed with gentle taps of the mallet.

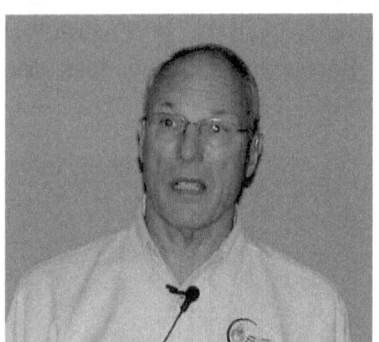

Lew Zirkle

The whole process of guided drilling, finding the slot in the nail and inserting the screws is simple and elegant. This makes First World standard of care for long bone fractures available all over the world. You don't even need electricity—even though it speeds up the process! I go over the process many times in the next few days until I've mastered it. Of course, real bone covered with real flesh on a real person will be different but I'm confident I can do it...*inshallah*.

SIGN was started 10 years ago by Lew Zirkle, an American orthopedist who has spent his life in developing countries. His mission is to provide the possibility for equality of fracture treatment around the world. By the end of 2008 SIGN had over 144 programs in 49 countries involving over 3000 surgeons who have performed over 36,000 operations.

Now, Tchad and the Béré Adventist Hospital will make it at least 50 countries. We have been given the instruments, our first set of 30 intramedullary nails, a cordless drill with sterile cover, training videos, wound suction treatment systems and the full support of the SIGN team.

Greg also gets a set for the Koza Adventist Hospital. We return to Africa better equipped to raise the standard of care in the poorest areas of the world.

27 August 2009
Copenhagen

Sarah and I are in Copenhagen visiting our friends, Henrik and Pernille. Sarah went to high school with Henrik and was in the same class as Henrik's little brother. They worked together as DJs at the school's radio station.

We've come again to Denmark for fertility treatments. It hasn't worked at all with our first doctor so now Sarah has us an appointment with Denmark's most experienced fertility specialist and one of the first to do IVF in the country. We just started the process last week in Aarhus.

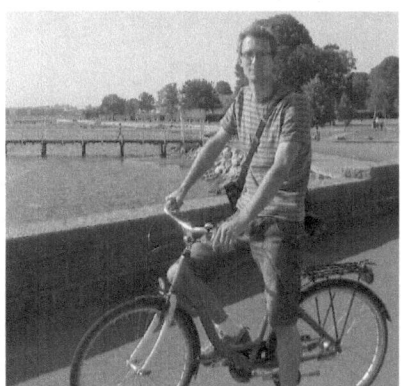

James

Today, we decide to go on a bike ride through the Danish capital. It's a beautiful summer day, the sun is shining and there's a cool sea breeze wafting through the streets. We rent bikes just down the street from Henrik's apartment near the central train station.

Copenhagen is biker friendly. There are separate bike lanes and even special bike traffic lights. We pedal through narrow streets in the shadow of old high rises. We glide around square ponds that were once part of the ancient moats protecting the city. Then we move out of town along the coast through Denmark's most prestigious neighborhood.

The houses, while impressive, would be just like a normal middle class neighborhood in the USA. This fits well with Denmark's egalitarian culture. What doesn't fit is our next destination: the royal hunting lodge. It's more like a palace than a lodge and is situated on hundreds of acres of forest filled with wild deer.

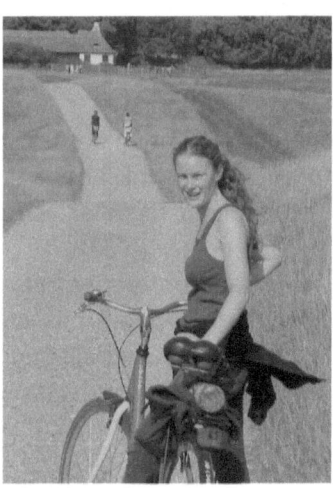

Sarah

The numerous bike paths are exhilarating and we fill our ravenous bellies with a wide variety of plums and apples just spilling over walls and falling to the pavement.

Finally, we reach our destination: the ADRA Denmark office. We meet with the director and describe what we are doing in Tchad. He offers to help us by sending a container of equipment.

The bike back to Copenhagen is leisurely as we are exhausted, but invigorated at the same time.

04 October 2009
Dancing

I start out by telling the story of a woman caught in adultery and brought before Jesus. That same woman later washed Jesus' feet with her tears at a dinner party. The young people around me seemed shocked at a God that would love that much. I went around and reluctantly got all of them to admit that God loved them just as much.

Then the festivities began.

Pierre's second oldest daughter and three friends get things off to a slow start. The younger girls are embarrassed to dance and the older girl is embarrassed to be dancing by herself. Amos then kicks things off in Nangjéré with a furious rendition of "*Kukusebur ne Jesu Christi*" as Tabitha rounds it up with a raised, twirling fist and a high pitched "*Ayyyee yi yi yi yiiiiiiiiii!*"

Several Tchadians sing a song in bad Nigerian English accompanied by a guitar. It falls flat. They redeem themselves by kicking up their heels and clapping their hands to an up beat French song accompanied by a tight but simple guitar staccato.

I then tell the story of the Samaritan woman who meets Jesus by Jacob's well. We are in front of a packed house. Samedi translates.

Suddenly, Samedi jumps to his feet. Daniel, a school teacher, has just gotten up to sing in his tribal language, Kera. The rhythm is catchy and many heads are bobbing. The drums are pounding and Samedi can't hold back any longer. His overweight, yet strong, body has lost it's flexibility as he stomps to the small group surrounding Daniel and raises his fist pumping into the air. He circles around with the inner foot pounding out the beat as his body weaves back and forth.

Bruno jumps up. The smallest of Pierre's boys, he stayed the same size since he was 13. Despite being almost 18, he still has that pre-teen look. His energetic body bounces up alongside Samedi. His knees bob up and down and both arms are raised.

Doulgue slides in smoothly stepping fluidly in and out of the dancing circle. The beat intensifies. Lam Daniel is whipping the drum as if it was a delinquent child. Allah lifts up his chin staring to the sky as his little hands flap in a furious blur all over the surface of his goat skin drum head. Koumakoy sets his drum down and hauls his lanky, athletic body across the aisle to join the fray, his shoulders bobbing up and down as his bent arms are held in closed fists against his chest.

Doulgue jumps up and looks directly at me. "It's not only Nangjéré that can sing Nangjéré songs. James, come here."

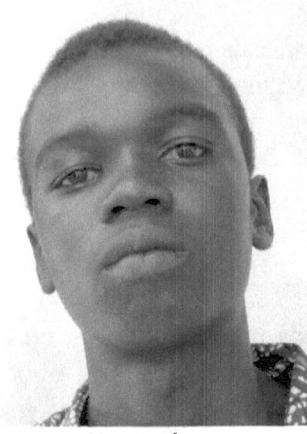

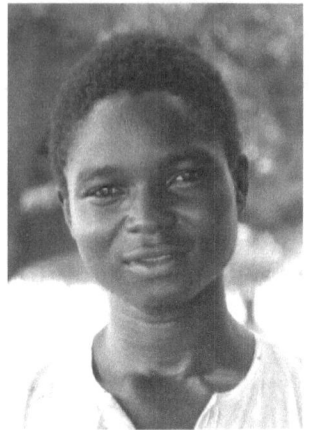

Koumakoy   **Doulgue**

Grinning from ear to ear, I stand up and walk over to him, my brightly colored matching pants and shirt swishing as I walk. I'm throughly loving the first truly spontaneous church service I've ever been a part of. Doulgue wants to sing his favorite song in Nangjéré. It's a song about Peter walking on water. We belt it out at the top of our lungs as Amos and a couple others join us.

I'm not much of a dancer but I find my head, shoulders, and legs unable to resist the pull of the rhythm. We finish strong to many a heartfelt *amen*. Degaulle's daughter stands up in the back, her baby hanging from her breast and lets out a high pitched wail. Antoinette echos from the back row of the choir. She keeps herself hidden shyly behind the kids in front, but she can't hide her smile. Tabitha finishes off the response with a piercing cry that can only be appreciated by those who have lived in an African village.

The dancing and singing goes on into the early afternoon, much later than usual. Group after group gets up to sing. We have sung in English, French, Nangjéré, Ngambai, and Kera. No one has understood everything, but everyone has been moved.

After lunch many of us, *Nasara* and Tchadians, head to the river. I climb the new bridge and stare down into the muddy, swirling water below. A crowd has gathered and I can't back down. I step up on the railing and launch myself out. My outstretched arms smack the water hard 30 feet below. The current quickly sweeps me under the bridge. I swim over to the support posts and find an eddy in the center. I rest briefly before striking out for the shore and clambering up the stony bank.

Back on the bridge, someone shouts out *"Lapia!"*

I turn and see Marty smiling in the midst of the crowd along the rail. Marty has spent many months at the Béré Adventist Hospital. In 2004 he survived a hippo attack but spent seven hours in surgery and four months recovering. The next year he was hospitalized for two months with tuberculosis. Now, he looks in perfect health.

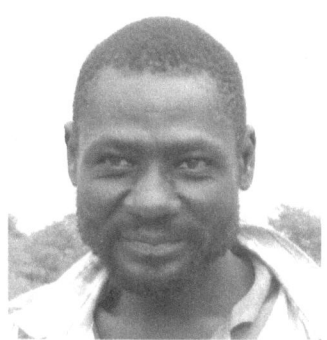

Hippo-bite Marty

I rush over and grab his hand with both of mine shaking it vigorously as I greet him in Nangjéré. I call Jamie and Tammy over.

"Hey, this is the guy in the documentary that was bitten by the hippo!"

Carson and Michelle come over. Tim and Melody join us as well. All the foreigners want to shake his hand.

"Marty is famous in the United States," I tell the crowd. "That's why all the *Nasara* want to greet him."

Everyone laughs as a local man translates my French into Nangjéré. As all the *Nasara* get their picture taken with Marty, I think how ironic this is.

Usually it's the foreigners who are the center of attention that everyone wants to stare at or greet. Now, it's a poor fisherman who just happens to have been bitten by a hippo right before a film student came to make a documentary of our hospital. The film won some awards and was shown all over in the Adventist Church in the USA and Denmark. Because of that film, many people gave money to support the hospital allowing it to become one of the best in Tchad.

I walk back over to Marty and the man who translated before.

"Tell Marty that getting bit by a hippo *was* a tragedy," I say. "However, God used that experience to help the hospital to become what it is today thanks to the film that he was in. Despite all he suffered, God turned it around to help many more people who are suffering."

As the man translates, Marty looks at me with a warm smile out of his small, bearded face. He nods and shakes my hand before walking off down the bridge.

04 October 2009
Plumbing

I stick my hand up the drain pipe. I want to clear out 30 years of accumulated debris, but I just can't get to it all. I manage to twist and angle my arm just right to get it in further. But now I can't get my arm out. I think I'm stuck. I start to panic. I twist and turn. Finally, scraping the skin off my knuckles on the rough cement, my dirty hand pops out.

Jamie and I are in Moundou redoing the plumbing for the new surgery center. Almost everything has needed to be replaced.

First thing we do is go to the local *Quincaillerie*. Everything that I thought I could never find in Tchad is stacked from floor to ceiling in a dusty, brick warehouse. We spend hours hunting down all we need. A large Arab in a simple white *jallabiya* and a well trimmed gray beard walks in. He is the owner, Mahamat.

"*As-salaamu aleikum,*" I greet him.

"*Wa aleikum as-salaam. Inta afé?*"

"*Afé, taybiin?*"

"*Al hamdullilah!*"

"*Mashallah!*"

The greetings over, Mahamat walks behind the counter. We continue shopping. After early afternoon prayers, Mahamat returns.

"*Vous...mangez...*" he starts in broken French and then switches over to Arabic. "We want you to eat with us. What do you think?"

He almost seems sure we'll refuse. He is pleasantly surprised by my profuse response.

"*Shukran, shukran*, it would be an honor, *shukran katiir.*"

He ushers us into a tiny side room under the overhead office built high in the corner of the warehouse. Mahamat sits us down and a huge platter is slung on the table before us. Piles of fluffy rice fill one huge bowl. A cast iron pot from Nigeria holds the steaming meat sauce. A shallow bowl to the side is bursting with a fresh tomato and onion salad.

Surprisingly, we are given spoons to eat with as generous portions are heaped into our bowls. Jamie, the vegetarian, digs right in, ripping the goat meat off the bones. Our host comes in last and there are no more chairs. We try to rise and give him ours, but he insists we remain seated. A special bowl of cumin flavored yogurt sauce is placed in front of him along with a plastic bag filled with fluffy flat bread the size of large crepes.

"*Bon appétit!*" Mahamat wishes us in French and grabs a pancake. He bunches the whole thing into his hand leaving the ragged edges pointing out. He mops up some yogurt sauce and shoves the whole mess into his mouth.

After gorging ourselves, we are all finally able to convince him that we can't eat any more. He reaches outside and pulls a plastic bottle of wild honey off the shelf. He dumps some more rice in a bowl and covers it with honey.

"*Faddal,*" he motions to me to dip in.

"*Adiil marra wahid!*" I say exuberantly, showing my pleasure.

I reach in for more, but he shakes his head and pulls the bowl over to himself. Then he motions to one of his workers to pour me some of my own. I can't figure out if he just wants to eat it all himself or doesn't want to have too much direct contact with an infidel. In any case, I finish the honey rice in no time.

Mahamat rises and thanks us again.

"The French are always too busy. The Chinese sometimes take a snack or something, but this is the first time I've eaten a meal with a client here in my shop. *Vraiment, merci beaucoup. Merci, merci, merci.*" He continues to thank us.

He is quite pleased and so are we to be honored in this way. We return to the job site.

I'm in the new operating room. Armed with Jamie's hammer drill I attack the floor. As the drill engages a puff of cement dust bursts out of the floor. When the bit hits the compacted earth beneath the slab, the dust turns red. I slip out the drill bit and put in the small chisel. I feel the vibrations all the way up my arm to my shoulder. The chirping of the chisel and the cracking of cement fills the room.

That night I sit on a hard stool under the stars in front of Antoine's house. The moon is three quarters' full and provides enough light to eat by. Antoine's wife serves us tiny, twisted potato-like tubers covered with cabbage and peanut sauce.

Antoine seems discouraged. The junior high that he runs has had a drop in enrollment. I try to encourage him.

The next day Jamie and I are back working at the clinic. Jamie attacks the bathroom. Meanwhile, the ladder I'm on is a little unsteady as I get to the top rung. There was no attic hole left in the new ceiling but one angle at the corner of the roof has been left open. I think I can squeeze through. I reach my hands up and grab the truss. I pull up as my feet kick out in mid air. I get to my waist and my tiny butt almost gets stuck but I slither through. I hop from truss to truss dragging the loops of plumbing pipe that I punch through the holes down to the sterilization room and consulting rooms below. The sweat makes the cobwebs stick to my body. I try not to fall through the fragile ceiling below.

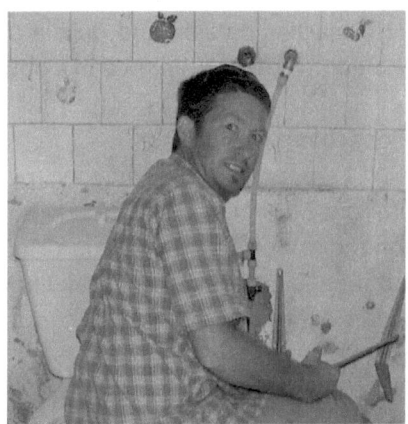

Jamie

We drive in to downtown for lunch. I pull the van up outside a brightly painted wooden shelter. There are cartoon images of fish, chicken and millet painted garishly on the corners. Inside a crowd is loosely seated around a selection of differently sized rickety tables and wobbly benches.

There is a tiny one open right in the middle. Someone, maybe a waiter, quickly wipes off the plastic mat covering the wood with his bare hand leaving a mixture of spilled beer and salad juice on the surface. Jamie and I sit down and nod hello to those sitting at other tables just a few inches from ours. Most seem to have liter bottles of Gala beer in various stages of consumption. The two men dressed in suits next to us are dipping their hands into a common bowl of lettuce and tomatoes covering some kind of meat.

"What's good to eat here?" I ask one of the men.

"Mutton ribs and salad's what we're having, *c'est tres bon!*"

"*Merci.*"

I order two servings from the overweight Tchadian woman in charge of the kitchen carved out of one corner of the room. The sounds of popping oil, the clatter of cast iron pots and the smells of wood fire smoke waft out from within.

A man approaches selling watches and cheap sunglasses. In the far corner, a man is stretching a piece of cloth between his hands to show a woman how strong it is. Several other women are looking on eagerly as they sip their beers. A large man who looks more Nigerian than Tchadian comes up behind me and holds out a package of medication over my shoulder and in front of my face. There is a picture of a smiling black man on a yellow and red backdrop with "Super King" emblazoned boldly across the front. In small letters underneath I see the generic name for what is known in other circles as Viagra. I turn to look at the man who raises his eyebrows and winks.

"Super King?"

"*Non, merci, je suis deja un Super King,*" I joke with him as I shake my head.

Disappointed he moves on to greener pastures.

Our meal has arrived. The cook holds out the traditional plastic basin with a plastic pitcher and brown soap for hand washing. I rip off pieces of tender, savory flesh off the sheep ribs, topping it off with lettuce, tomato and onion drenched in a vinaigrette. A small pile of grilled yellow chilies adds some spice to the mix. I wash it all down with some Top pineapple soda and then help Jamie finish off the last of his meat.

10 October 2009
Mahamat

I usually get annoyed, but this time I decide to make a game out of it. I'm sitting in a borrowed car in front of a hardware store. On the other side of the street is the Grand Central Mosque of N'Djamena. It's hot. Sweat drips down the back of my *jallabiya*. I haven't been drinking enough water. I just met with Mahamat Saleh and Aimé to talk more about the project in Abeche. Mahamat Saleh gave me a copy of the papers for the land the government has given us: six hectares. Sarah and I then spent some time with Pastor Etienne at the mission office and a few hours in the market.

Now, I'm leaning out the window staring in the face of two young, ragged-looking Arab boys. They hold out the familiar metal bowls on a string and quote verses from the Koran. They are asking for *zakat,* one of the five pillars of Islam. Instead of just replying with *"Allah eftah,"* I start to speak to them in Arabic.

"Kikef? Inta afé?"

"Afé."

"Mashallah! Usumak yatu?"

"Ana Mahamat," says one.

"Wa ana Abdoulaye," says the other.

Mahamat and Abdoulaye are now grinning shyly from ear to ear. The hands holding the metal bowls have dropped to their sides. I hold out the half full can of apple soda I've been drinking.

"Dorah charib?"

Mahamat eagerly holds out his hand and takes a swig. Abdoulaye shakes his head and backs away slightly. I take another sip and again offer it to Abdoulaye who again politely refuses. I give the rest to Mahamat and they both walk a few feet away and lean against the back of a parked Land Cruiser. Several other boys come up in ragged robes with their own metal bowls in tow.

"As-salaamu aleikum!" I greet them and again ask their names.

By this time, an older boy on crutches has approached. He's about 15 and has a skimpy turban wrapped around his forehead leaving the top of his head bare. He speaks a little French. The other boys rattle off their names:

"Mahamat!"

"Hissein!"

"Mahamat!"

The older boy smiles and says that he is also called Mahamat. I look down at his leg and see a bulge under his trousers on the left lower side. I also smell the distinct odor of a packed third world hospital.

"Can I see your leg?" I ask the older Mahamat in French.

He pulls up his pants revealing two stainless steel bars suspended above his tibia by seven pins sticking out of the bone and skin surrounded by a dirty, Betadine soaked gauze wrap. His foot is swollen. I unwrap the gauze and see pus coming out from around the pin sites. Apparently, a car hit Mahamat six months ago. The driver of the car took him to the hospital, paid for his surgery and then disappeared. Since then, Mahamat hasn't had the money to go back to see the surgeon.

By this time a crowd has gathered. I explain to the crowd that I'd like to help the boy if he can come to Béré. A retired soldier walking with a limp and a cane suggests I go find Mahamat's parents. Sarah walks out of the hardware store with some cans of paint. We load the car. Sarah climbs in the back and I help Mahamat into the front seat.

I follow the road encircling the Central Mosque and Mahamat points down a side streets. We leave the pavement and start bumping over the rain ravaged dirt roads that still make up most of the Tchadian capital's thoroughfares. I turn right and then left. Mahamat waves out the window at an old man sitting on a mat in front of a a mud wall.

"Abbah, as-salaamu aleikum!" The old man waves back like a beauty queen on a float.

We turn down an alley and pull up in front of a small mosque jutting almost into the road. Robed and turbaned men are streaming out after the afternoon prayer. We stop in front of a tiny, wizened man selling cucumbers piled haphazardly in a mound on a tattered mat. It's Mahamat's father. I step out as the crowd flowing from the mosque circles up around us. Sarah stays in the back seat.

"As-salaamu aleikum!"

"Wa aleikum as-salaam!"

"Kef halek?"

"Afé, taybiin?"

"Mashallah!"

"Baraka!"

"Al hamdullilah!"

The staccato greetings ring out. I shake Mahamat's fathers hand and Mahamat points out his mother, a burly woman with no neck and a chubby face surrounded by a black head scarf.

Someone is sent to bring Mahamat's x-rays. I hold them up to the light. They are the originals showing a compound fracture of his mid-tibia. I give him money to pay for new x-rays in the morning. A woman completely cocooned in a green, sequined body and head wrap becomes the spokesperson. She speaks excellent French. I get her number as well as the number of another neighbor and promise to call as soon as our van is repaired and ready to go back to Béré. Sarah and I will take public transport back to the hospital in the morning.

I turn to Mahamat sitting in front of his father. Mahamat has unwrapped his head and has a happy grin on his face. I address the dad.

"Tamam sahi? Are you in agreement with what I say?" The old man nods and smiles. His wife agrees to accompany her son to the hospital.

I climb back in the front seat and wave good bye. The phone rings.

"Hello?"

"Yeah, this is Rivers," says a voice in English. "Listen, we have a sick baby here. The family we're living with, one of the patriarch's wives just gave birth a month ago and the baby has a fever of 103 degrees Fahrenheit. What should we do?"

"I think I should see the child."

"Ok, we'll meet you at TEAM in an hour."

I have to return the borrowed car, so Rivers follows me from TEAM to Sara and David's house. Sarah and I had spent the night there after castrating Sara's horse.

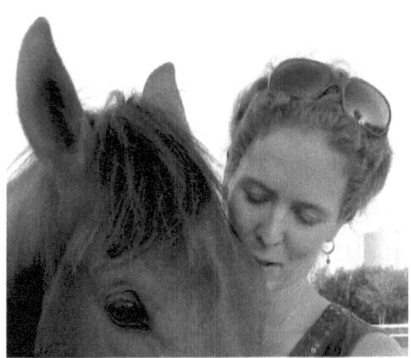

Sara the Swede

Sarah and Sara had become friends after meeting in church one Sunday at the Bible Translator's compound. Sarah is Danish and Sara is Swedish. Both are thin with red curly hair and love horses. Needless to say they hit it off right away. Sara had wanted her horse castrated for months but couldn't find a vet willing to do it. Horses here in Tchad rarely if ever gelded. We promised to do it a long time ago but now we got the chance.

I drop off Sara and David's car, thank them and get in Rivers' small station wagon. We drive through the back streets of N'Djamena and pull up in front of a large gate. In the front courtyard, a group of men are playing cards on a mat. Rivers greets them in Goran. I do the ritual in Arabic. We follow a side path to the back of the house where we find the women also sitting on mats under a straw covered shelter. The baby is lying in front of a young woman with bright eyes, a colorful dress and beautiful head scarf.

I kneel and examine the child. She is tiny and breathing fast. Her heart is racing and she looks a little pale. I suspect malaria and tell the mom she needs to be treated right away or she may die. The mother starts sobbing hysterically throwing herself into the arms of the women beside her. The man accompanying shakes his head and smiles. Rivers takes me back to the mission guest house. I write out a reference paper with the treatment I feel the baby should have and sign and seal it with my rubber stamp.

Just then, Odei pulls up on his motorcycle.

"*As-salaamu aleikum!* Are you ready to eat?"

"Are both Sarah and I going to ride on the *moto*?"

"Impossible, there's a problem with the back tire. You'll have to take public transport."

Just then, our van limps into the compound. She blew a head gasket on road to N'Djamena the day before. By adding water every 20 minutes and leaving the radiator cap loose we managed to hobble into town. A new volunteer from the USA, David jumps down, adds water and tosses me the keys. Sarah and I follow Odei's motorbike. It's a dark night in dimly lit N'Djamena. It starts to rain.

We bounce along over rutted out roads out to the suburbs of Farcha. There is no electricity out here. We pull up in front of a tiny hut. It is dimly lit with the warm light of a kerosene lamp and the cold blue of a battery powered halogen table lamp.

A rickety wood table supports a huge platter with eight or ten covered dishes. Another smaller platter has two clear plastic pitchers and six upside down glasses with the word *Lemon* written on the sides. One pitcher has the deep purple of Hibiscus flower juice and the other the burnt yellow of a strong ginger drink.

There is a small bench behind the table where Sarah and I sit. Across from us are three chairs for Odei, his wife Rachel and his older brother. The ceiling is made of rice bags painted with orange and dark green Arabic designs. The walls have an electric clock that chimes on the hour, a large photo of Odei's wife, and a calendar.

Rachel brings out many courses: potato, carrot and tomato salad; fried potatoes covered in mayonnaise vinaigrette; rice and pasta with chicken in tomato sauce. Sarah and I haven't eaten much since breakfast and the feast settles in nicely. We rinse it all down with many glassfuls of sweet Hibiscus and biting ginger juices.

I tell Odei that his uncle is doing fine. We took out his infected kidney on Monday. It was inflamed and stuck to everything. The nurse called me last night to say he's drinking milk and wants to eat. In N'Djamena, the urologist was asking $1400 for the surgery. We did it for $150.

We are sad to say goodbye after such a pleasant evening. Sarah is glad to crash when we get back to the guest house. I pick up a volunteer from the airport before I finally sink into my mattress and let the coolness of the fan whisk me off into dreamland.

19 October 2009
Drained

I'm drained. Literally. Yesterday morning they took one bag of blood. Last night they took another. I know your not supposed to give blood more than once every three months. But I couldn't help it. I didn't want to live with any regrets.

It starts yesterday on rounds. Michelle comes up and asks all the nurses rounding with me what their blood type is. She's looking for someone with B negative blood. No one has it. She forgets to ask me.

"Aren't you going to ask me what my blood type is?"

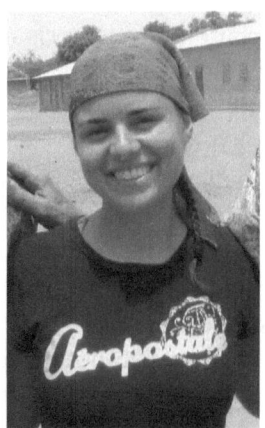

Michelle

Michelle looks at me and says sarcastically, "What's your blood type, James?"

"B negative," I reply.

"Really, do you want to give? We've been looking all morning. None of the family members or staff has the right type. It's a small child with a hemoglobin of 2.2."

"Ok, no problem. After rounds."

I continue rounds. I can't write because for the last two days my index finger has developed a red angry bump on it. It started as a small pustule that I ruptured with a needle. I got some pus out, but since then, it's gotten bigger and more painful. I've been on antibiotics for two days with no improvement. I probably should lance it, but am a little afraid. The last time I incised an abscess on my body I had a non-healing tropical ulcer for almost a year. But it's so painful I can't even hold a pen to write. The nurses write out my orders and I finish rounds.

After rounds, I go to my office. Matthieu kneels down beside the exam table I'm resting on. I look at the ceiling, waiting. I feel a sharp sting as the 14 gauge needle pierces my left antecubital fossa. I squeeze the spongy ball in my hand to make the blood drain out quicker. I continue to stare at the ceiling. Finally, Matthieu pulls out the needle and I look at the bag filled with dark red, B negative blood. I've never even seen the child I'm hoping this blood will save. I jump up, feeling no ill effects of draining off 1/2 a liter of blood.

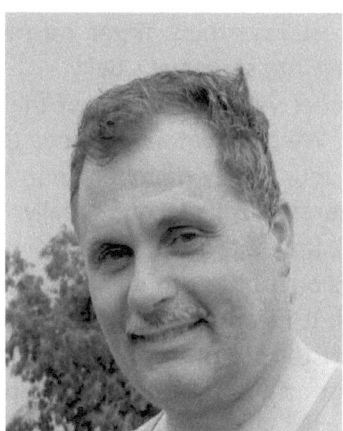

Tim

I've had to cancel all surgeries because of my finger. I should really drain it. I call Dr. Tim who has offered to give me a finger block. He prepares the local anesthetic in my office. I feel the needle try to pierce my skin. The needle pushes down hard before finally piercing through.

"You've got tough skin." Tim comments.

He injects the Lidocaine slowly so it doesn't sting so much. Then he repeats it on the other side of my finger. My finger becomes like a piece of dead wood. It's eery. I touch it with my other hand. I have the weird sensation of feeling in one place where I should be feeling in two.

I try to pick up a pen, but it just seems weird even though I am able to hold it normally. I pull out the scalpel blade. As I lay it on the red skin I feel a little nervous. But I don't feel I thing, so I insert it through the top of the inflamed area. Dark blood pools out but no pus. I dig deeper and find some thick yellow stuff. I twirl the scalpel inside the wound and more pus comes out. It's drained at last.

I pack and wrap the wound and go back to see the ER patients. I finish early since there were no operations. I go home and rest.

In the late afternoon I go back to the hospital and see Tim in my office doing an ultrasound on a young girl. Based on her history I suspect appendicitis. But then I see the scar on her lower abdomen.

"She was operated on here by you last year," the girl's father says.

I look through the *carnet* and see that I took out her appendix. I look at the ultrasound images. There's free fluid in her abdomen. Her belly is swollen and very tender. She needs another operation.

I call in Abel and Siméon. I go home to get a bandaid to seal up my finger wound. An open cut on a finger is high risk during a surgery. I hope I can use it. It's the most important finger on my body, especially for delicate tasks like cutting into someone's belly.

I return to the hospital. Abel comes out of the OR and says the girl's hemoglobin is 6.7 g/dl. We call Anatole. He finds that her blood type is B negative. He tests the four family members with her and none of them can give. I decide to operate anyway. I don't really want to drain my blood a second time within 12 hours.

Dark red fluid surges out of the abdominal wound along with a mass of blackened small bowel. It has twisted on itself from an adhesion due to her last surgery. I untwist it but most of it is already dead all the way to the large intestine. I cut off the dead part, sew up the hole in the colon and reattach the proximal end to another hole I make in the cecum.

My finger is stiff and I can't tie the sutures well so I have to do instrument ties for everything. Her heart rate stays at about 140-160/min through the whole surgery despite two large bore IVs running full blast. At least her initial hypotension soon resolves. She needs blood.

As I close up the skin, a penetrating thought enters my head. *If she dies overnight and you haven't given her your blood, won't you regret it wondering if that small red gift might have saved her life?* I call Anatole.

He's checked two more family members without success. We go to my office.

The needle goes in again. Same arm, slightly different vein. This time I feel a little weak afterwards. One liter drained. I sit on the bed for 15 minutes before slowly walking home. I drink a liter of cold Gatorade that Sarah has prepared. It helps a lot. I get home and crash. I'm completely drained.

01 November 2009
Ultrasound

Sarah has missed her period. We did IVF again in Denmark two months ago and now she has missed her period for sure. I'm a little nervous as I turn on the ultrasound machine. We've been disappointed too many times already.

The machine whirs on and I squeeze the cold gel on Sarah's lower abdomen. I apply the probe and press down into her pelvis. Slowly my eyes adjust to the static picture of the ultrasound. Can it be? I move the probe around and confirm the presence of an embryo in the uterus. I even find a heartbeat.

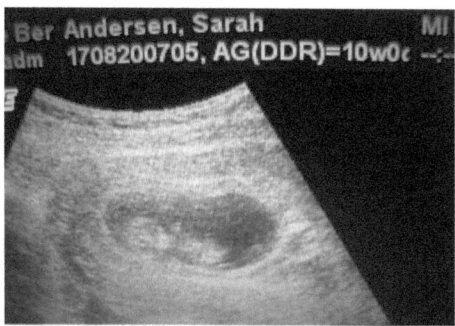

Ultrasound of Sarah's first pregnancy

I look at Sarah with tears in my eyes but a wide grin on my face. She smiles back. I take a picture and print it out. We go home hand in hand.

It almost seems too good to be true.

04 November 2009
Euthanasia

"The pain started suddenly at 4 o'clock this morning," says the man stretched out before me on the gurney. He is in obvious distress. His abdomen is swollen and he's gasping for air. I look at his carnet. His name is Gaouna.

"How was he yesterday? Was he sick at all?" I ask through his brother who interprets from French to Ngambai and back again.

"Yeah, yesterday he was fine, but this morning, the pain started right here," he points to the epigastric region of the patient.

I examine the belly. It's firm but not tense. When I tap with my fingers it sounds hollow, full of air. Gaouna winces in pain with each touch: peritoneal signs. His breathing is shallow and his heart is rapid and his pulse weak. It sounds like a perforated ulcer.

The ER started an IV already. I tell Abel to give Gaouna triple antibiotics and call in Samedi from home. I go see the last of the ER patients. Meanwhile the OR staff preps for an immediate laparotomy.

The family doesn't have money to pay. However, they are well to do and leave their motorcycle at the hospital as collateral for future payment.

I finish in the ER and come back to the operating theater. I enter the room. Gaouna is lying on the OR table. Two IVs of Ringer's Lactate are raised high on IV poles running in fast into both arms. A foley catheter has about 300mL of dark urine. His arms are stretched out on the arm boards and tied down as if he's about to be crucified.

Gaouna's eyes are closed and his breathing is even shallower and more rapid. The beep of the pulse oximeter tells me instantly he's not getting enough oxygen. I glance at the numbers. He's at 60% saturation, way below the accepted norm. I'm afraid Gaouna is not going to make it. Maybe we're too late.

We have no oxygen, so I decide to intubate him. I grab a cardboard box off a top shelf. Inside is a mix of all our endotracheal tubes. I select one I think will work. I test the cuff with a 10cc syringe of air while Abel pulls out the laryngoscopes.

In my hurry I forget to prepare suction or put in a stylet.

I check the laryngoscope and the light works. Abel injects 2mL of ketamine and I insert the blade in the Gaouna's mouth. The light isn't working. I pull it out and give it a tap. Nothing. I take the blade off and put it back on the laryngoscope handle. It works again.

I put the instrument back in his mouth and lift up the tongue. I briefly see the vocal cords before a mass of saliva obscures my view. I call for suction and try to put in the breathing tube anyway. It bends down away from the vocal cords.

I reach behind me and quickly leaf through a drawer in the anesthesia cart to find a stylet for the tube. I slide the stylet into the ET tube. I bend it into a distal hook to help me put the tube into the trachea. I try again and this time am successful. I attache an Ambu bag to the tube after blowing up the cuff and start to breathe for our dying patient. His saturation comes up to 85%. I give the bagging over to Abel and go scrub. Samedi and Abel have already prepped and draped the abdomen. I'm sure that with release of the abdominal tension, Gaouna's breathing will improve.

I take the large scalpel and am quickly in the abdomen as a surge of dark red, slimy fluid surges out. Samedi quickly suctions out over 3 liters of fluid. The intestines look injected and angry but don't seem to be gangrenous. I start to explore and soon discover the real problem. As I open up the abdominal wall to expose more of the contents a purplish, lumpy, alien-looking mass pops out of the right upper quadrant.

Gaouna has end-stage liver cancer.

Inside I'm furious. As I quickly try to close up the useless operation, many thoughts whirl through my head. *How could the family deceive us? Of course, Gaouna's been sick for months if not years. Without CAT scans and other diagnostic equipment we base so much of our diagnosis on history and physical exam. This surgery could've been avoided. Now in all likelihood he'll die before making it out of surgery. How could God have let me make such a big mistake costing so much money for Gaouna's family and so much time and personnel resources for the hospital?*

I've never closed up a surgery quicker. I take the Ambu bag off the breathing tube. Gaouna's sats go down to 57%, but stabilize as he starts breathing on his own. I just want to get him out of here alive. I take out the ET tube. We transfer Gaouna to the gurney and wheel him out to the wards. I explain the prognosis to the one family member who's there.

An hour later, Pierre comes to inform me that Gaouna has *rendu l'ame* (given up his spirit). I'm not surprised. By this time, I've had more time to reflect.

What if we wouldn't have operated? Gaouna may have lived several more days or even weeks. But he would've suffered. We have no real good pain medication. In the hospital, we can give IV pentazocine, but it's not that great. And the pain pills we have, Ibuprofen and Paracetamol, wouldn't have done much. By operating on Gaouna, we let him slip away in a Ketamine coma without any suffering. Sure, the operation didn't save his life, it just saved him from a torturous death. So was it the right decision after all?

06 November 2009
Poop

Silently and stealthily, the man slips through the shadows of a dark Tchadian night. The Béré Adventist Hospital has become his temporary domain. His child is hospitalized for severe malaria. A blood transfusion is slowly dripping life back into his boy's fever wracked body. The man has sinister motives. He really needs to take a dump...

The hospital has had trouble for years with patients relieving themselves in piles on the ground in the tradition of the African bush. Despite the availability of latrines, the smell and foreignness of the cement structures is revolting to someone used to the pleasant peacefulness of natural surroundings of soft grass or sand. In the 1990's, a resourceful night watchman named Jairus made successful war on the perpetrators. He would take the pile of excrement in a rubber gloved hand and move from bed to bed. He would wipe some of the stool on each bed until someone confessed or turned in the guilty party. They then had to go out and bury the leftover turds.

The problem only got worse with the building of a fence around the hospital in 2004.

Now, this evening, maybe the tide will turn. Our unknown man makes his way quietly past the operating theater to the outside water faucet. Taking a comfortable position squatting, the man flexes and stretches his thigh muscles. He pulls down his pants and reaches out to get a firm grip on the metal water pipe coming out of the cement slab. This is his chosen receptacle.

Suffering from a common Tchadian ailment, his knuckles turn white as he strains to force out the poop hardened in his dehydrated and constipated colon. A sigh of relief accompanies the success of his mission until a bright light suddenly blinds him.

A harsh cry of *"Ca c'est quoi?!!"* brings an end to his devious deed.

Literally caught with his pants down the man hurriedly tries to cover his naked manhood. Jean-Jacques, our vigilant gatekeeper, hauls him roughly to his feet. Even though it's a little after midnight, our new administrator, Augustin, comes immediately from home.

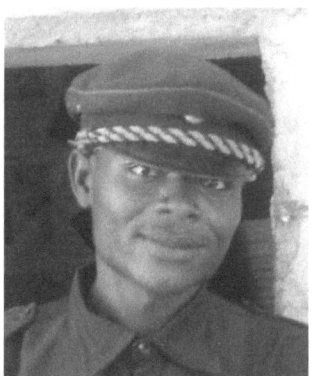

Jean-Jacques

Punishment is swift. Augustin calls the gendarmes. They force the man to pick up his caca and stuff it in his pocket. Then the gendarmes escort him off to prison. He was last seen weeding the flower garden in front of the jail.

16 November 2009

Games Tchadians Play

The woman is in the OR for emergency surgery. Sarah comes to inform me that the family has only paid 15,000 CFA of the 25,000 CFA required.

"Wait here," I tell Samedi and Abel. "I'll see about that."

I slip off my OR shoes, put on my Crocs, slide my mask down my face, push open the screen door and put my game face on.

A beacon of light comes out of the pharmacy window in an otherwise dark ad building. As I approach, I see a tall, lanky Tchadian in dark tan matching pants and short-sleeved button down shirt. He slowly turns at the noise of my entrance and looks me up and down. His face is familiar. He's one of the former teachers at our elementary school. His name is Amos.

I can tell he's sizing me up. Let the games begin.

I march up to Amos. "What's the meaning of this?" I sputter with a look of disdain on my face. "I hear you haven't paid for the surgery yet!"

"What do you mean?" Amos looks at me with a shocked and hurt look on his face. "I've just paid 10,000 CFA."

I look at the pharmacist, Koumabas, who nods with his goofy half grin. He's enjoying the match.

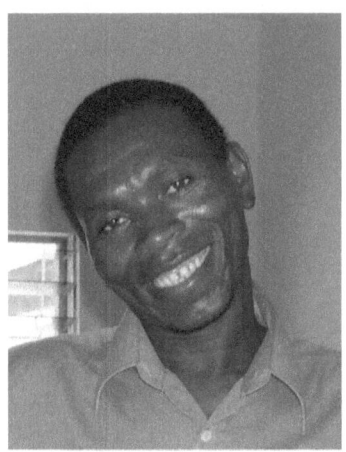

Koumabas

I turn back to Amos. "Do you realize that you should pay 25,000 CFA?" I ask in feigned disgust. "Do you think 10,000 is equal to 25,000? Aren't you a teacher? That's basic math!"

"*Pas de problème,*" Amos responds coolly without blinking. "I'll just pay the rest tomorrow. Go ahead and do the surgery. You can trust me."

"Everyone says that," I laugh. "But we've found that if they don't pay before the surgery they never pay after. Find a solution!"

I pretend to turn away.

"But we're different," cries Amos. "Maybe other people don't pay, but we will. You know us."

"Yes, I do," I retort. "That's why you need to pay ahead of time. Look, we want to save your sister's life. We're ready to operate. We're only waiting on you!"

I've played my trump card. Out of the corner of my eye I see Koumabas nod approvingly. He's enjoying this immensely.

"*Ok, ça va, ça va,*" Amos pretends to concede defeat. "I have my bicycle outside. Can I just leave that as collateral to prove I'll pay later?"

"Let's see it."

Amos soon returns dragging in a rusty, bent and twisted carcass of a bike with missing pedals and a torn up seat.

Here it is," Amos smiles smugly, sure he's won.

Koumabas just shakes his head and chuckles. "*Ça la!* No way. That's worth 10,000 CFA at best! That's not enough!"

I've found a tag team partner in this traditional Tchadian sport.

I narrow my eyes, fixing them on Amos. "Don't you have a cell phone? You could leave that as collateral as well and then we can get going on saving your sister's life. We're only waiting on you, you know!"

"I don't have a cell phone," Amos looks shocked. "I'm just a poor teacher." He looks like a puppy with his tail between his legs begging for bread at the table.

It's all I can do to turn away, but I've got to finish the game.

"Oh well, I guess we'll just have to wait," I shrug. "We're all ready and everything. Just waiting on you."

I fold my arms across my chest and lean casually against the wall.

"Ok, ok," Amos starts to lose his composure. "David, come quickly!"

Our night watchman comes in and extends his hand towards Amos holding a tiny cell phone in his outstretched palm.

"David, is that yours?" I ask. I don't want Amos to cop out by forcing our staff to cover for him. I won't lose that easily.

"No, no. It's mine," Amos doesn't even blink at the outright lie he just told me. But then again, I haven't exactly been telling the whole truth either.

"Thanks, Amos, you did the right thing." As I turn to leave I stop and look back.

"By the way, I've already done my part," I say with a smile. "We've finished the operation, the ovarian mass is out. She's doing fine, we just kept her in the OR until you paid. Too bad I had to play this game to get you to do your part."

02 December 2009

Perforation

It must be bad. They only call me out of church for real emergencies. I gather my books and walk out on the dusty dirt floor to a bright late Tchadian morning. Noel and Pierre are waiting for me. I don't see a nurse anywhere. What's going on?

"Abel's in-laws have just informed him that his fiancee will come to him tonight to become his wife. He has nothing to prepare a wedding with but wonders if we'll do a dedication for him in church."

After much discussion it is decided that the women of the church will prepare a goat that I will provide and we'll do a wedding ceremony at his house tomorrow evening. He has no family here, so we will be his family.

That afternoon, I'm too tired to go to the river. It's a good thing as Tchibtchang soon comes calling with the traditional *clap-clap* of the hands instead of a knock at my door.

"There's a father who brought his son in for a blood transfusion for severe anemia and malaria. After we drew his blood to give to his child, he told us his hernia popped out as he was riding a motorcycle on the way here. We can't get it back in."

I accompany him to the hospital and see Siméon and Abel already waiting.

"Aren't you supposed to be preparing to welcome your bride tonight?"

Abel chuckles loudly with a huge, toothy grin. "No, tonight she comes to my house, but I'm not supposed to be there until tomorrow night...so here I am!"

A quick look reveals that this hernia is not going to be reduced without surgery.

Just then Augustin One comes in. "There's a guy who's been gored in the butt by a bull."

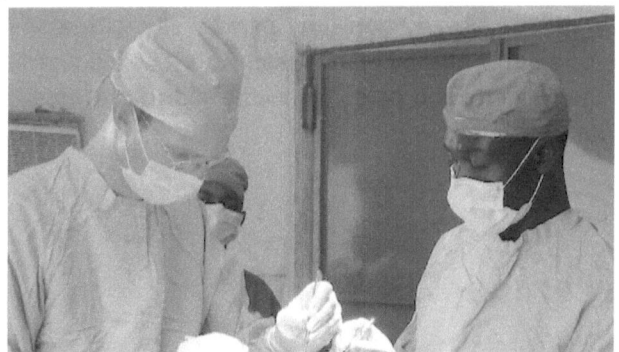

James, Siméon & Abel

"Ok, bring him over here." When he arrives, I take a look. Fortunately the gore wound is to the side and back of the anus missing the intestines. It's pretty deep, though, so I order antibiotics. Meanwhile, Siméon and Abel have been preparing for the hernia.

Siméon gives the spinal anesthetic while Abel scrubs. I prep the surgical field with Betadine and then scrub. Abel puts my gown on and snaps my gloves into place. A few scalpel strokes later and we see a dark mass of intestines. I open the hernia sack and there is already some dark, coagulated blood in the mesentery but the intestines still look viable. I push the squishy, slippery mass of bowel back into the abdomen and close the hole. He also has a hydrocele. I check to make sure his left testicle is good before taking out the hydrocele on the right, testicle and all. I sew a piece of mosquito net over the weak spot in the muscle and close the skin.

The man with the anal wound is stoic. I give him local anesthesia and close the wound in four layers leaving the skin loosely approximated. I tell him to soak in salt baths four times a day and go home.

Later that evening, Augustin One asks me to see a little girl who was treated here a month ago for malaria. She now has a swollen belly. I approach her bed on the pediatric ward and see a thin little six year old with bright eyes who looks tired but not too acutely ill. Her belly seems slightly swollen but is soft and non-tender. She has diarrhea, so I put her on Chloramphenicol and Metronidazole and go home.

The next day, Sunday, I lazily do rounds around noon. Melodie asks me to see a girl on pediatrics she feels isn't doing well. Her glucose is a little low but she's awake. She just doesn't want to eat. It's the same girl I saw last night. She is alert but refuses to eat. The diarrhea has all but stopped but her belly seems more swollen.

I examine her and the belly is soft and she doesn't flinch or anything when I touch her. I look in her face and something in her gaze tells me there's something serious going on. I feel a strong impression that I should operate on her. I feel bad because this means I'll probably miss Abel's wedding. I tell the father and he agrees. Koumabas calls in Siméon and Samedi.

When I arrive in the OR, Samedi has already scrubbed. The little girl is lying resignedly on the operating table. I feel a sudden panic. *Why am I operating on her? Maybe she has abdominal TB.* I run to my office and bring in the portable ultrasound. The images reveal a full bladder and a lot of stool but no intra-abdominal fluid. Well at least it's not abdominal TB. I'm still uncertain but feel committed now to the operation. I scrub and join Samedi at the surgical field.

We all bow our heads and I pray in French *"Dieu, we're not sure what's going on with this girl. We just pray we are doing the right thing. Help this operation to be a success and this little girl to recover her health completely afterwards."

I cut through the skin and fascia below the belly button. The peritoneum seems thickened and I'm not sure if the intestine is stuck. I enlarge the incision to above the belly button and make it into the abdominal cavity. A gush of liquid stool spurts out under pressure as we try to suck it up. At first, I'm afraid I've punctured the bowel. But as the stool spills everywhere over the surgical drapes I soon see that she must have had a perforated intestine. I can't believe she didn't have pain but am relieved we decided to operate.

Samedi sucks out the stool as we irrigate and search for the damaged section. My finger digs into an inflammatory mass and a clump of green, peat moss looking stool slithers out. We've found the hole. I pull out the mass, clamp and cut it out. It's in the distal ileum. I then suture the two parts of good intestine back together, rinse out the belly with liters of fluid, put in two drains and close the fascia and partially close the skin.

It's 5:00pm when we finish. Sarah and I go home and change clothes then walk across town with Jamie, Tammy, Abre and Siméon. The sun is going down and a full moon is half-way risen. The village of Béré is relatively quiet. There are no electric lights ruining the mood. A few people walk home from the market. An ox cart creaks as it comes back from the fields bearing rice straw. Children run up and down, wave and scream *"Lapia, Nasara!"*

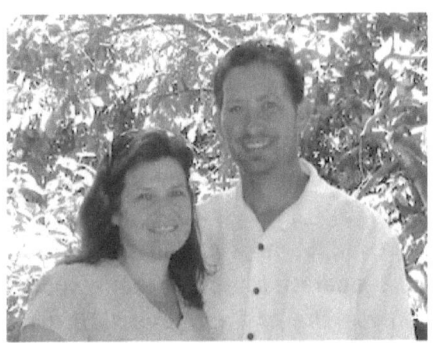

Tammy & Jamie

We enter a courtyard where plastic chairs have been set up under a tree for the family of the bride. In front of them are three chairs for the officiants: Noel, Degaulle and Gueltir, dressed for the occasion in dark suits. Facing them across a plastic table with a Bible and a cheap flashlight are Abel and his bride. Abel is wearing designer jeans and a nice, short sleeved, button down shirt. The bride is decked out in a traditional dress with matching head scarf stylishly tied off in an impossible way as only an African woman can do.

I sit down on the ground behind the couple, next to the kids and Pathfinders sprawled out on mats. Pierre motions Sarah and I over and we are given plastic chairs behind Noel. I was supposed to give the wedding speech but Noel is covering for me and amazingly is saying almost exactly what I had planned on saying. I relax. Noel finishes and then turns to me.

"Now, Dr. James will give advice to the couple."

I start to panic. All I've prepared has already been said. Fortunately, the choir has also gotten up thinking it's their turn. I motion for them to go ahead while I quickly look up some verses in the Bible with the help of a flashlight. The whole wedding is now only lit by the full moon and a single, battery powered halogen lamp on the table in front of Noel.

The choir is swaying and dancing to a catching, rhythmic song about the importance of marriage. I speak a few words about how important forgiveness is in marriage and then the choir sings some more. Noel stands up and announces that the couple can now embrace. Abel looks shy and awkward but the bride saves the day by turning to him, grabbing him by both shoulders and pulling him towards her as she bobs from side to side kissing both his cheeks. The crowd erupts in applause and cheering.

Some of the men bring out tables covered with huge pots of boiled goat sauce, rice and homemade onion rings. Noel's wife, Achta, comes by with a basin and a plastic pitcher so we can wash our hands. Conversation and laughter flows freely as the food is devoured. Abel's new father-in-law gives the closing prayer.

Sarah and I walk slowly home in the moonlight, my hand on her barely noticeable pregnant belly. Two small girls swing happily holding Sarah's hand. A small boy runs up to me and grabs my hand. We all go merrily home with the final songs of the choir fading out behind us in the distance.

13 December 2009

Premature

I try to think happy thoughts. I focus on the pleasant sounds of the African night. But, no matter what, I can't sleep. The pounding of the drums keeps me awake. It's not the simple happy rhythm of the children singing silly songs in the moon light, but a deep, dark, forbidding thumping accompanied by mournful howling. It sends chills down my spine and into my guts. It leaves me feeling ugly and used. I'm forced to put in earplugs.

The earplugs help too much. The next thing I know, Sarah is tugging me awake. I struggle out of the deepness of a pleasant unconsciousness into the darkness and chill of an early Tchadian morning. It's 3:30am and Samedi is at the door. I stumble over to the screen while pulling on an old pair of scrub pants.

"*Oui?*"

"*Docteur*, there's a woman referred from the health center. She's seven months pregnant and bleeding. Her skirt is soaked in blood but her vital signs are stable for the moment."

"Ok, start an IV, give her Ampicillin, place a foley and prepare her for a C-section. Call Siméon and Abel. Oh, and give her 10mg of Dexamethasone IM, first thing. Call me when she's ready."

Earplugs back in, I'm soon back in La-la Land. This time my slumber is not as profound. It's as if something from my conscious is trying to break through. I wonder why I'm still sleeping. *Why haven't they come to get me*? I get up and pull on a scrub shirt to go with the pants I'm still wearing. It's 5:00am. I walk up to the hospital as the first light of dawn barely illuminates my path through the mango trees and over the sand covered in horse dung. Even from a distance I can see the lights in the OR are on.

I arrive and the woman is still in the delivery room. We bring her to the OR, turn on the generator and Samedi scrubs while I shave and prep the abdomen. After a spinal anesthetic, the woman is placed supine and I scrub as well. I say a short prayer and then take the large scalpel blade. I cut into her abdomen through the fascia and tear the muscle and peritoneum apart to get to the uterus. After deflecting the bladder away, I nick the uterus with the scalpel and push a curved clamp inside releasing a fountain of clear amniotic fluid. As suspected, she has a placenta previa. The placenta covers the exit from the uterus and starts to bleed profusely when labor starts.

I reach my hand inside the uterus and find a tiny little head way high above the placenta. Samedi pushes and the tiny, premature infant slips into the world. She grimaces and flexes her arms and legs. Her skin is underdeveloped and translucent, revealing all her underlying blood vessels.

Samedi clamps the cord, I cut it and we hand the little girl to Abel. We soon here a shrill little scream as the girl opens her lungs to that life giving oxygen. As I suture the uterus closed, I have Abel turn off the fan in the OR and cover the baby up. We have no baby warmer and I'm afraid she'll get cold.

I finish sewing up the skin and take of my gown. We clean up the blood and mess around the woman and I go see the newborn.

She's cold and has a slow heart beat. I pump her chest a few times and the heart beat comes back up. I put a tube in her nose and give her some sugar water. I have Abel go tell the family to boil some water. We'll heat her up that way.

Meanwhile I pick up the tiny form that fits easily in my two hands and place her naked body against my stomach under my shirt. I'll use my own body heat to warm her. After a few minutes I feel a response. She starts to move more and make some weak cries. I pull out the feeding tube and suction out her mouth and nose since she's regurgitated some of the sugar water. I feel her stretch her tiny feet against my belly. Her hands are grasping. She's reflexively searching for her mother's milk. I curl her up in a ball and hold her close flipping her around like a burger on the grill to make sure she gets cooked on both sides.

I go out to check on the hot water several times. Each time, the family says that it's ready, but it never is. Finally, I can't wait. The morning chill is too much. I take her home, held tight against me under my flimsy scrub shirt covered with a woman's wrap the family gave me.

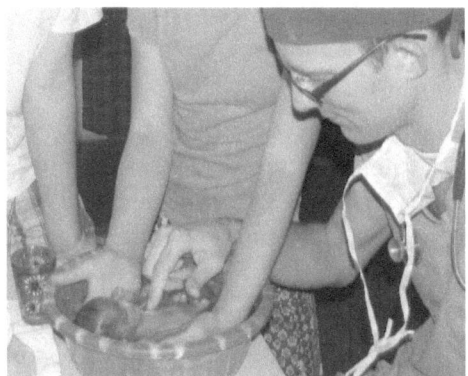

Cory, Brichelle, James & premie

I knock on Tammy and Jamie's door. Tammy lets me in. I explain the situation and Tammy quickly heats up water as Cory and Brichelle come to help. We put hot, but not scalding water in a plastic basin and put the girl in. She seems to like it and kicks and stretches. She's breathing well and has a strong heartbeat. Her limbs are quickly warmed up as we replenish the hot water supply. I gently hold her head up so her mouth and nose stay in the air to gulp down that important oxygen.

Tammy prepares some warm water with sugar and we let her suck a few drops from a tiny syringe which she gingerly swallows. Cory and Brichelle are fascinated by the perfection of her tiny fingers, toes and whole body. She opens her eyes and looks at us as if to say thanks. I can't help but think of the tiny baby inside Sarah that is only a few months younger and developing quickly.

Suddenly, she regurgitates again and stops breathing. I try to clean out her airway with the syringe and start chest compressions. She rapidly turns pale and starts to get cold. Every once in a while she makes a desperate gasp. Her heartbeat is almost negligible. After 15 minutes of CPR I give up, wrap her in her cloth and silently walk through the chilly desert morning to give her back to her family.

Death has struck again.

22 December 2009

Excuses

This has been one of my worst days yet. Believe me, I've had my share of bad days. But this definitely ranks (as in stinks) up there with the "best" of them.

I could find plenty of excuses for my behavior. For example, we've done more surgeries the last 3 weeks than the last 2 months combined—including one 7 day stretch where we did 46 major operations. I could cite the fact that over the weekend I've had amebic dysentery for the first time. For the last three days I've been nauseated, anorexic, fatigued and generally miserable.

But I'm tired of excuses, that's all I hear all day long and that's what started this day off so badly.

"Enock left at six without giving sign-out," says the day shift nurse. "But he said he HAD to go to Kélo."

"We don't know why the kid didn't get his blood transfusion," adds the pediatric nurse. "Enock left for Kélo and didn't tell us."

"The father left four days ago," interjects the child's mother. "He said he'd be back with provisions and to donate his blood, but he hasn't come back. Can we go home now?"

"Madame, your child has a hemoglobin of 3.3," I reply patronizingly. "He'll die if he doesn't get that blood, besides you've already paid for it anyway and the father has the same blood type."

"But he's gone home. It's far away. We have no money."

"Madame, do I need to remind you that you don't have to pay anything and we'll find one of our staff to give?"

"But my husband isn't here, he went home to...." I cut her off in mid-sentence. Michelle gives blood and soon the child is on his way back to health.

"I don't know why this guy's still in the ER," says the ER nurse. "I wasn't the one who hospitalized him four days ago."

"Haven't you had a night shift and a couple of ER shifts since then?" I query. "You just let him stay even though his wounds were sutured and they weren't severe enough for him to need to be hospitalized? What about his relative who was also beat up who didn't even need sutures? He's also occupied a bed for four days in the ER."

The two patients had been beaten up because they tried to steal rice When the owner of the rice tried to stop them they cut off his arm. So the relatives attacked them and they ended up in our ER now for four days. As I tell them they have to leave the hospital now, they start muttering under their breath.

"YOU didn't do anything for us! Four days in the hospital and nothing!"

"What about the four wounds we sutured closed and the pills that you have been taking?" I ask.

"But we didn't get any IVs or shots or anything. Next time, we're going to the hospital in Lai!"

"Doctor," shouts another nurse running up. "This patient is writhing in pain!"

"I have his *carnet* here for an ultrasound," I respond. "I'll get to him when I can."

"But he's really in bad shape! Come see him."

I go outside. A barefoot man covered in dust is standing calmly to the side. I walk him over to the ER where I can examine him. I look in the *carnet*, nothing written in it except "abdominal pain." The plan is to have him see the doctor and get an ultrasound.

"Ok, let's find out more about his pain," I tell the nurse.

I start to ask questions, but none of the nurses know his dialect. They call in a translator who starts translating. It's an excruciatingly slow process. I'm frustrated and walk out yelling over my shoulders.

"Find out all you can about his pain and then come see me!"

Somehow, before I can even get back to my office to do other ultrasounds, Sarah is there to present me with the same man's *carnet*. The nurse had managed to stop doing what I asked him to do, get ahead of me, find Sarah and give her the carnet...all before I could walk the short distance from the ER to my office.

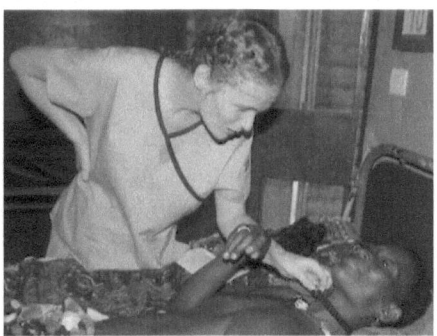

Sarah & patient

I storm back yelling at anyone and everyone in my path. I'm totally out of control. I spend most of the rest of the day yelling, shouting, flailing my arms, insulting people and making a fool of myself.

The nurse calls me back to the ER to see a man with abdominal pain for five days. He hasn't pooped in five days either. He hasn't vomited. He ate some porridge yesterday, but didn't feel like it today. He's lying comfortably on the bed. Sounds like constipation to me, a real problem here. He has a fever so probably has malaria as well. I tell the nurse to prescribe quinine and treat his constipation. As I'm about to move on a small urging tells me to examine him more closely. I can't explain why. A still, small voice perhaps.

I bend over him. His belly doesn't look too swollen. He has no findings that you wouldn't expect from constipation. If he had a bowel obstruction or appendicitis he would've been vomiting by now after five days. I push and tap some more. He's somewhat tender, but doesn't seem to have peritoneal signs. I'm still not satisfied. Something inside says that my initial impression is wrong. I get a glove and do a rectal exam. He's more tender on the right side than the left. Maybe he does have something.

I decide to operate.

Sarah calls me when the spinal has been done. Samedi and Abel have scrubbed and draped the patient.

I enter the OR and notice a pool of yellow fluid on the right side of the patient next to the OR table on the floor.

"What's that?" I ask.

"Maybe his foley has come out," says Sarah.

Samedi lifts up the sterile drape so we can look. I pull back instinctively as I see a huge puddle of liquid stool with floaters between his legs. It's been dripping down the drape to the ground.

"Well, I guess it was constipation after all! Looks like the relaxation from the spinal was all he needed."

I turn to walk out of the OR. Again, I sense something deep within, something that has almost been repressed from my full day of self-righteous, angry behavior. That little something makes me turn around and go back in.

"Well, since he's already anesthetized and prepped, we might as well have a quick look around inside his belly."

"*C'est bon,*" Samedi nods in agreement. I go and scrub.

As I open the belly, nothing jumps out immediately. The intestines aren't swollen or inflamed. There's no rush of blood, pus or fluid. I start to poke around inside. I look for the appendix on the right. I can't find it. Everything looks ok...suddenly, out gushes some thick pus. I open the incision for better exposure and peel away the inflamed bowel. With a scoop and a flick of my index finger, the ugly looking appendix pops into the surgical field. An obvious perforation is at it's tip.

I remove the appendix, irrigate and aspirate the abdomen, place a drain and close up.

I spend the rest of the afternoon and evening listening to the night shift team bombard me with questions about things the morning team didn't do or follow up on. I go see two patients that have wounds that don't want to heal. They keep having stool come out of places it shouldn't. I'm at a loss as to what to do for them.

Later, I pass hours in the prep room with Samedi, Sarah, Abel and Abre searching for IV access on two infants with anemia needing blood transfusions. I spend most of the time yelling and throwing things as I can't find the vein and can't thread the catheter when I do. Finally, Samedi gets the last one in.

"Halleluia!" I shout and try to go home.

As I close up my office, Rosine is there looking at me sweetly as she innocently asks, "Can you help us find an IV? We've been searching all afternoon and the kid needs blood..."

"Don't bother me," I snarl. "That's not my specialty. I don't find IVs very well. That's nurses work. Go find someone else and whatever you do, don't call me!"

I go home. As I walk through the door, I pause. Sobs begin to wrack my body. I am filled with anger that wants to explode right out of me. I don't want it but it's there. I feel betrayed, overwhelmed and extremely ashamed of my behavior today.

Yet, in spite of it all, somehow God spoke to me. He made me save a man's life instead of relying on my own skills. I would've sent a man with a perforated appendicitis home to die with a couple of laxatives to go.

I think I'll ask for forgiveness tomorrow.

04 January 2010
Homemade

"There's a guy in the ER with what looks like a bullet sticking out of his face." Franklin tells me casually, as if commenting on the weather.

"A bullet? Is he stable?" I question.

"Oh yeah, he's fully conscious, sitting up, talking. He walked in. Apparently he was hunting and the rifle backfired or something and the bullet went into his right cheek. He came from quite a distance. I think it even may have happened yesterday...my French isn't that good."

"But it's not too emergent?"

"No, I think it can wait."

I am happy to hear that, since we are working on our eighth surgery of the day already. It has been quite the Monday. Samedi did some hernias and hydroceles while I did rounds. Then I did a prostatectomy and a hysterectomy. Now I'm putting an intramedullary SIGN nail in the tibia of a man who had a motorcycle accident 10 days ago and just now comes in. He'd been sutured up in a health center and then sent home for traditional bone setting. Now he came in with a mushy, floppy, foul smelling lower left leg with shattered, exposed bone in the center. It looks like the infection hit the fascia and marched up his leg to behind his knee with skin eaten up and the underlying flesh putrid and rotting.

I'm tempted to amputate. However, after debriding the wound, it looks clean and has good blood supply all around. About 10 cm of bone is exposed but I figure if it was my leg I'd want someone to try and save it no matter how slim the chances.

So I reset the exposed bones easily and hold them in place with bone clamps. Then I incise the knee down to the tibia, insert the bone awl and ream out the bone marrow. After selecting the size of intramedullary nail I attach the external guide arm and twist and hammer the rod through the center of the broken bone. I then use the other guides to drill through the bone, find the hole in the rod, and place the fixating screws. After swathing the raw flesh in diluted bleach soaked gauze, I wrap the leg in an Ace wrap and send him off to the recovery room.

Meanwhile, I've been called to the ER for a strangulated hernia. Sure enough, the huge scrotal hernia won't reduce so we take him urgently to the OR. Fortunately, the dark intestine pinks up when freed up from it's strangulation. There is a lot of blood tinged inflammatory fluid so I leave in a drain and order post-op antibiotics and IV fluids.

Finally, it's time for the bullet. The man is wheeled in on the gurney. He is fully awake and cooperative. The right side of his face is covered with a compress and some tape surrounding a blunt metal spike that looks like the tip of a bullet sticking a couple centimeters out of his right cheek next to his nose.

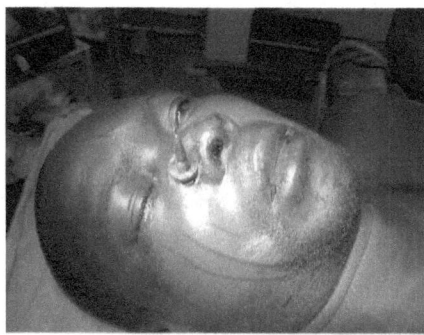

Franklin puts him under with Ketamine and I start to explore. I grab the metal point with a strong clamp, it doesn't budge. It twists some, but doesn't move. I take a scalpel and incise around the foreign body down to the cheek bone. I grab and twist some more. A spring surrounding the spike pops up and out of the skin. *What is this?*

I probe deeper. The cheek bone is shattered at the entrance point. I push in a little and sense something soft and jello like...his brain. He also has cerebrospinal fluid coming out his nose which confirms that this thing is deep. I twist, tug, rock, rattle, jiggle and any other movement you can think of. The object won't move. The only thing I know now is that it isn't a bullet.

I slip a hemostat down beside it and it seems there is a thicker piece at the end of the shaft that is behind the cheek bone blocking it from coming out. Finally, by levering it down to poke the thick piece up higher and then wiggling and pulling at the same time the projectile pulls free. I pack the wound as deep and gently as I dare and examine the object.

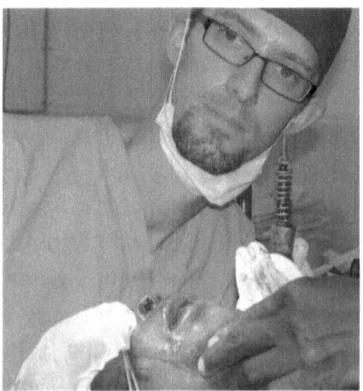

James & firing pin

Samedi laughs and says he recognizes it now. It's part of a locally made firing mechanism for a homemade rifle made right here in Bere. The man had been out hunting with it and it misfired sending the cheaply welded, spring loaded firing pin into his cheek, past his sinuses and into his skull touching his brain. That explains the burn marks on his right hand and around the gaping hole in his cheek.

We move him off to the hospital wards and I slowly walk home through the cool, dry desert evening with only the stars to light my way.

17 January 2010

Dinah

I feel her kick for the first time. I've felt other fetuses kick before on other pregnant women's bellies, but this time is special. The child is mine. A thrill goes through me and a silly grin wraps around my face. It's Friday evening, Sarah has malaria and I've just started her treatment with IV Quinine. Leaving Sarah, who wants to rest, I go spend some time with Franklin and boast about my strong, athletic little daughter. After a little singing and worship, I return home.

After checking the IV drip with a flashlight and being satisfied it's running well, I crawl into bed and fall fast asleep.

A gentle shaking startles me from a profound slumber. My heart sinks at Sarah's words.

"I'm all wet down there, what could it be?"

I try to reason that maybe it's urine, but my heart tells me differently. Her bag of water has broke. The pregnancy is only 21 weeks, too early too survive if she delivers now.

I pull on some shorts, grab a flashlight and head up to the hospital. I bring back the portable ultrasound. I place the jelly on her belly and confirm my deepest suspicions: our little daughter has almost no amniotic fluid around her. However, her heart is still beating normally and she is still kicking if not screaming. I take the ultrasound back, but halfway there realize I've left my keys at home. After making the return trip, I pick up my obstetrical textbook and try to find the pertinent passages.

It's not encouraging. Most women with preterm rupture of membranes and fluid leaking deliver in less than two weeks and the outcomes are not good. I take the book home and discuss the bad news with Sarah. We pray, then try and sleep. We both toss and turn all night long. Drums pound in the distance as someone in the village seems to be mourning a lost loved one. Sarah has just a little more leaking through the night and by morning it seems to have stopped.

It's Saturday morning. I give Sarah some yoghurt, hang up some more IV fluids and head out to church at 8:30am. The doors are shut. It's a cool desert morning, but the sun is starting to heat things up. I sit in the shade along the rough brick wall in the dust. I'm reading a little when I sense a presence beside me. I look up. A tall, poorly dressed man stands proudly to my right clutching a tattered Bible. As he greets me I recognize him as the husband of one of our patients who explained to me yesterday that he's a traditional healer from up north.

We start talking. I soon discover he is a man of God if not a prophet. He can barely speak French, but his words have a power that can only come from above. I confide in him and ask him to pray for Sarah and my unborn daughter. My spirits are uplifted.

After the teaching in the first part of the service, I head home to check up on Sarah. She's vomiting and not feeling good. I stay with her. I look back at the passages in my obstetrical book and see a section saying that if there is at least one pocket more than two centimeters deep, than the outcomes are surprisingly better. I go back, get the ultrasound and to my joy find a three centimeter pocket and another two centimeter pocket. The heart still beats well. Maybe there is hope that Sarah won't lose the pregnancy.

We start to plan. If Sarah hasn't delivered in two weeks we'll change our plane tickets and head to Denmark. That way we'll arrive when the baby is 24 weeks and has a chance of living with modern intensive care nursing.

We rest all afternoon as I try to control Sarah's nausea and treat her malaria.

She starts to have contractions that night. Some bloody discharge discourages us again. I sleep only fitfully. When I wake up, Sarah informs me the contractions stopped halfway through the night. I repeat and ultrasound and our girl is doing fine, if anything it seems like there is more fluid inside.

Hope rises...then falls as the contractions start again after breakfast. Sarah is in agony. She is moaning and tossing in pain. She vomits frequently. I try anything and everything to control the pain and vomiting. Nothing works.

I am at her side almost constantly. She grasps my arms in vice grips every time the contractions hit. They are getting closer and closer together. She has more bleeding. I'm afraid, but repeat the ultrasound. The baby's heart is still beating well.

But then a contraction hits and I see the heart beat start to slow. I'm losing it. It seems almost to disappear, then miraculously, as the contraction ceases, the heart slowly picks back up. She's suffering. Her heart can't take much more. The cervix is opening. It's just a matter of time.

I prepare some towels and basins. I have a bottle of water handy. We start to talk of what to do with the body. Where will we bury it and what will we use as a coffin. Our conversation is interrupted every couple of minutes by severe pain and writhing as I sit helplessly by watching my wife suffer, knowing the outcome of her suffering will be an extreme loss. There's nothing I can do but be with her.

The cervix is dilating. I can feel our daughter's bottom. She is coming out breech. A few more contractions and Sarah cries out.

"She's coming!"

I reach inside and touch the tiny leg and foot. I grasp and gently pull as my daughter enters a world she'll never know. Her heart is still beating under my fingers. She fits in the palm of my hand. Every part of her is perfect. There are no malformations.

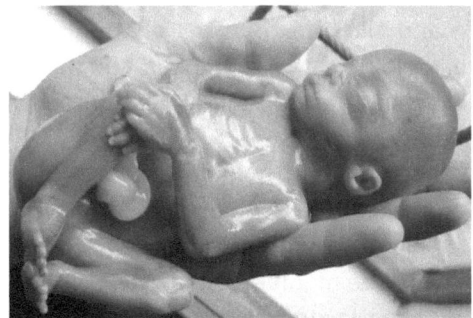
Dinah

She has Sarah's nose and my long skinny legs and arms. Her mouth is open as she tries to get air into her undeveloped lungs which will never be able to extract the oxygen she so desperately needs. Her little ears will never hear. Her closed eyes will never open. Her heart starts to slow down. But as I touch her tiny hand, she curves her fingers in an attempt to grasp my gigantic finger. She does this several times. She is getting colder.

It's all over.

I burst into uncontrollable sobbing. I hold her and watch her and examine her every little perfect human part over and over. We take pictures. Sarah lays her on her stomach. While she can curl up into the tiniest ball, when she's stretched out she's way longer than I could've imagined.

We wash her, tie off the umbilical cord and cut off the placenta. I place her in an old mayonnaise jar and seal the lid tightly. I dig a hole under the small tree with the red flowers just outside our door. The dry soil is rock hard. I use the hose to wet and loosen the dirt. I get down about two feet and bury our girl in the soft mud. Sarah shovels in the first few piles and I finish. I read from I Thessalonians 4 about the resurrection. Then I place a huge, porous stone over the top of the little grave as a marker.

Sarah has one thing to add, "Let's call her Dinah." I nod numbly. It is finished.

27 January 2010
Zakouma

It's a cool night in the Sahel. Baboons are howling across the wadi. I pull on my beanie and climb in the back of the modified Land Cruiser. Cutting off the cab, welding chairs in the bed and painting it forest green have made the old rebel attack pickup almost unrecognizable in its new role as safari-mobile.

I stand behind the front seat holding onto the bar across my chest. Gary fires up the engine and Wendy hands me the spotlight plugged into the cigarette lighter. Sarah is seated to my right and Cherise lays across Wendy's lap staring into the moonlit sky.

Gary and Wendy have invited us out here as a sort of retreat as we mourn the loss of Dinah and they continue to mourn the loss of Kaleb. The common tragedy of losing children has given us a strange sort of bond, a bond of shared sorrow and loss.

Except for a group of Tunisian engineers who arrived earlier in the evening, we are the only visitors to the Zakouma National Park near Am Timan. Exhausted by their 15 hour trip to the park, the Tunisians hole up in the restaurant, leaving us alone to explore the African night.

In a few minutes we have left the small campground behind and turn on the road towards the airstrip. To our right, a pool of water houses a couple of crocodiles. An image from earlier in the day flashes across my mind: a large jaw and head bursting out of the calm waters clutching a mammoth catfish temporarily in its teeth before twisting and swallowing the huge mouthful and disappearing again into the green depths.

We are looking for eyes. Skimming the spotlight across the tall grasses and acacia trees from right to left, we seek out the night prowlers and resting herds through the reflection of their eyes.

Groups of reddish green pairs reveal striped antelopes with twisted horns as triangular faces stare us down. Smaller reflections lead to tiny nimble footed gazelles that skip and hop and jump about, frightened by their own shadows. Narrow set eyes close to the ground on closer inspection lead to long, slender genet cats with their striped bushy tails hunting mice and other critters in the short grass around the watering holes as the slither and slink close to the ground. Large, bouncing eyes high in trees let us know of the presence of Galapagos tree climbers that are too swift to follow, appearing and disappearing only to reappear several meters away up the branches.

In the vast, green pastures around the water holes that dot the wadi, herds of gazelles, deer and antelope rest, graze and cast a nonchalant look at the passing human intruders. One herd is guarded by a pair of greenish, blue eyes, wide set apart encircled by horns flowing over the sides of the head like a wig over powerful shoulders and the stocky body of a cape buffalo.

Several hundred meters further on a group of those evil, green eyes is staring at us from the edge of the pond. Without a working four wheel drive, we are loathe to pursue. Instead, these fearless creatures make their move towards us as they huddle together and move confidently and deliberately towards the truck in an oblique maneuver meant to impress but not threaten.

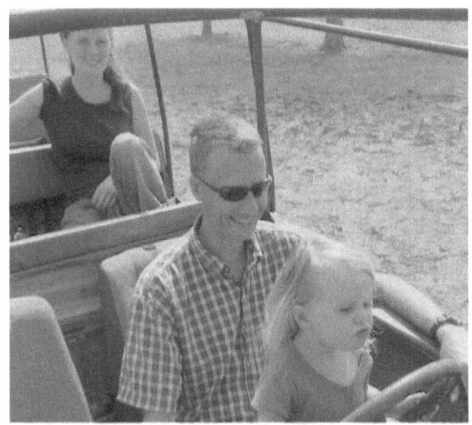

Sarah, Gary & Cherise

Huge black and white storks stand awkwardly in the marshes. Great herons balance on slender legs before taking off in lumbering flight. Small headed, spotted birds that fly like butterflies startle up from the road at the approach of the headlights. Some seem paralyzed till the last minute when they make a desperate flutter to escape right in front of the charging grill. Gary actually stops once and manages to get his hands around one that I've stunned with the spotlight before it flaps out of his palms.

Small, big-eyed birds reflect the spotlight like wild cats' eyes which temporarily confuses me until the eyes start to take flight. An owl stares us down with it's unblinking eyes sitting on a branch directly overhead before taking off, its silent wings beating noiselessly through the dry and dusty night.

Gary punches the gas and the Land Cruiser lurches forward. We move towards some antelopes grazing near the road and a dark, compact, lumbering creature holding close to the ground. He enters the road and turns, looking directly into our headlights revealing short, powerful legs and dense, black fur. A long, thick neck leads to a flattened head with a mouse grasped firmly in it's teeth. If there was still any doubt, its characteristic back and forth lumbering gait gives it away as a badger.

We get glimpses here and there in the distance across the grass of a larger, slinkier striped mammal: the African civet. A raccoon like tail disappears into the bush. A panther like back end slinks around a corner. We never get a full few, but enough to appreciate the grace of this medium sized feline-like animal.

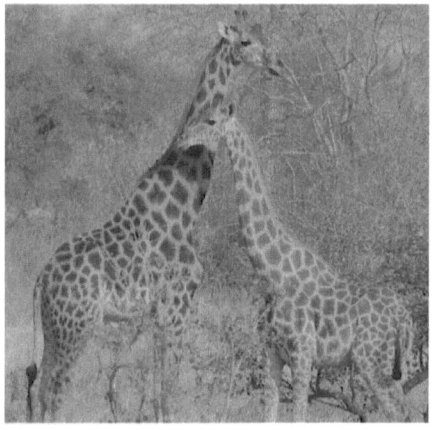

We see quite a few giraffes from a distance, but none up close. One small herd has a couple of babies only recognizable that far away by the reflections of the eyes being so much closer to the ground than the adults.

We near the end of our night safari. We pass the mud, thatched roofed huts of the village of Zakouma and pull onto the airstrip where Gary zig zags across at high speed. We see one hyena lazily reclining on the edge of the strip.

Coming back out from the hangar we see another Galapagos' eyes bouncing quickly away in the treetops. Back on the airstrip we see a group of eyes far away. We pursue and find two groups of four hyenas each, all lying down in two piles. As we pull within 20 feet, they rise up staring at us with evil eyes and panting jaws open revealing dangerous teeth over their skulking, spotted bodies. They move off into the bush, cackling in their high pitched witches' laughs.

At the end of the airstrip we take the road heading back to the camp. Out of the corner of my eye I see a big shape rise up out of the darkness. I swing the spotlight and just catch a giraffe who has just pulled to its feet ten meters away. Another giant turns its long neck around to stare at us from it's long face. Then, both amble gracefully away like a couple of long-legged models strutting their stuff.

They move up to a blob on the ground with a chimney pointing to the sky. Rocking forward to get it's hind legs up and then backward like a camel the slumbering giraffe gracefully and rapidly regains its footing. Picking up speed, the three now gallop off in seemingly slow motion, their front legs moving like huge scissors as their back legs move in tandem to catch up. They effortlessly cover huge amounts of ground in each stride. After putting a little distance between them and us they move back into their most graceful of walks like a couple of movie stars exiting the premier in their fur coats.

Several hundred meters later I briefly catch a glimpse of a large, black animal staring straight at me. I'm sure it's a baby elephant! Gary backs up and tells me to turn off the spotlight as it may charge. When we're just across from where I saw it, Gary plugs in the spotlight and we see a huge cape buffalo staring us down. Impressive, but not what I hoped to see!

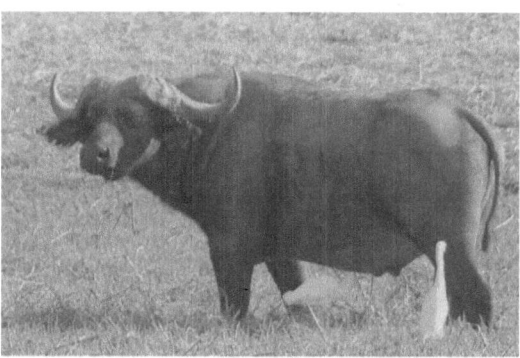

Almost back to camp, we see what looks at first like a dog running on the road ahead of us. We approach and when we are within a few feet it turns sharply into the bush. It's a Serval cat with a tiny head, spotted body and long, lithe legs and tail. It springs away as only a cat can and disappears into the night.

Just 100 feet from the turnoff into the camp I spot three pairs of eyes to the left. One pair lifts up revealing a blood stained snout. I shout at Gary and he screeches to a halt and backs up. We turn off the road and head straight for a recently killed buck. It's lifeless eyes stare back at us from the ground. Matted grass spills out from its stomach which has been left under a tree. The body is about ten feet away from the stomach.

Two hyenas lift their snouts out of the carcass revealing red stained fur all the way down their chests. The back leg is missing leaving a mound of tattered flesh up to the open abdomen pooled with blood. The neck shows no injury, but matted fur suggests maybe a lion killed it before being chased off by the hyenas. There are a couple more hyenas who slink around in the periphery of our headlights waiting for us to leave which we soon do.

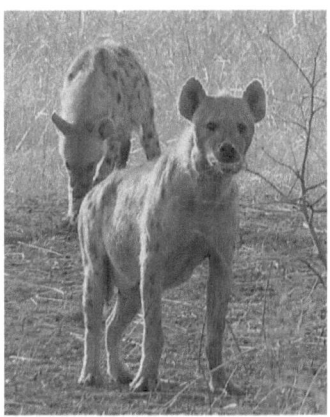

The next morning, we drive out to the site and see four hyenas fighting over all that's left: a piece of torn leather skin. Their bellies are engorged so they can barely walk. No bones, organs or even blood remains, only that tattered hide and the pile of grass that was in the stomach. One hyena tries to make off with the hide. Another runs up and grabs it. They engage in a macabre game of tug of war as they run off cackling and chortling into the early dawn...

The dawn of a new day in Tchad.

To be continued...

Glossary

Al hamdullilah: Arabic for "Praise be to God." Used often in greetings especially in response to queries about one's health.

Allah eftah: Arabic "God will make an opening" literally but has the sense of "God will provide." Spoken when one doesn't want to give alms, or *zakat.*

Ambu bag: Also called a bag valve mask, a manual resuscitator or self-inflating bag. It is a hand-held device commonly used to provide positive pressure ventilation to patients who are not breathing or not breathing adequately.

Anti-retroviral (ARV): medication to treat HIV/AIDS by slowing down the multiplication of the virus. To be most effective, three different ARV medications are taken simultaneously. ARVs can control AIDS but not cure it.

As-salaamu Aleikum: Traditional Muslim greeting, Arabic "Peace be unto you." The standard response is *"Wa aleikum as-salaam"*

Ascites: liquid in the abdominal cavity, usually from cirrhosis, (scarring) of the liver or cancer; in the developing world is often caused by tuberculosis

Bactrim: cheap, but effective broad spectrum antibiotic of the Sulfa class.

Baraka: Arabic "Blessing," very much sought after in Muslim culture.

Béré: village of approximately 15,000 in southern Tchad where the Béré Adventist Hospital is located

Béré Adventist Hospital: District hospital in Tchad's health care system founded by the Seventh-day Adventist Church in the late 1970's where the stories in this book take place

Betadine: Povidine Iodine, a brown disinfectant used to prepare skin for surgical procedures

Bouillie: traditional Tchadian porridge made of flour, rice, sugar, peanut paste and lime

Boule: traditional paste made with rice, millet, sorghum or corn flour boiled and then cooled in a half a calabash to make a half dome shape that is then taken off in pieces and dipped in a variety of sauces

Breech: The position of a fetus in the uterus, butt first, feet and head following; carries a higher risk for complications during delivery

Carnet: French word for small book. Portable medical record in the health care system of Tchad; usually made out of a school notebook cut in half.

Chai: Arabic "tea," a ubiquitous drink in Tchad for Muslims and non-Muslims alike. Taken very sweet with lots of refined sugar.

Chari: Main river in Tchad, joins with the Logone River at N'Djamena and empties into Lake Tchad.

C-section: Short for Cesarean section, a common obstetrical operation where the surgeon opens up the uterus through the abdominal wall to deliver the baby as rapidly and safely as possible. Reserved for complicated labor and delivery.

Debridement, to debride: Surgical term for cutting away dead tissue in an infected wound to speed up healing or arrest the advancement of the infection.

Diclofenac: non-steroidal anti-inflammatory medication that can be given orally or intramuscularly. Same class of medication as Ibuprofen and Naproxen.

Ectopic pregnancy: Pregnancy outside of the normal location in the uterus.

ER: Emergency Room.

ET tube: Endotracheal tube, a specific type of tracheal tube that is nearly always inserted through the mouth (orotracheal) or nose (nasotracheal), protects the airway and facilitates artificial respiration.

Plasmodium falciparum: most virulent strain of Malaria responsible for most of the deaths and severe complications of this global pandemic, also the most common and most drug-resistant species of Malaria.

Flagyl: anti-infective medication with a wide range of uses in treating tropical diseases such as anaerobic bacterial infections and parasitic infections such as amebiasis and giardiasis.

CFA: Central African Franc, currency used in *Tchad* and throughout francophone Central Africa, 500 CFA is equivalent to approximately one US dollar.

Fulani: Nomadic cattle herders ranging across most of western, sub-Saharan Africa, almost 100% Muslim. Also called *Peul, Fula, Mbororo.*

Ibliss: Arabic "the Devil."

Injil: Arabic "gospel," one of the holy books mentioned by name in the Qur'an. Refers not only to the Christian Gospels (Matthew, Mark, Luke and John) but to the entire New Testament.

Insan: Arabic for "mankind," from the root word *nas* meaning people

Inshallah: Arabic "if Allah wills or wishes."

IV: Intravenous, inside the vein, how to get medications and fluids directly into a person's blood circulation

Jallabiya: Arabic word for long, loose-fitting robe with long sleeves and matching pants, the most common garment worn by Muslim men in *Tchad*

Ketamine: anesthetic medication providing a dissociative effect allowing the patient to be operated on without pain, yet without losing his airway, breathing or gag reflexes; not used much in developed countries due to emergence reactions which can cause vivid nightmares and hallucinations.

Lapia: Greeting in *Nangjéré,* the local dialect of Béré; literally "health".

Mashallah: Arabic "whatever Allah wills."

Meconium: Newborn's first stool; if the meconium comes out before birth, it is a sign that the fetus is stressed.

Nangjéré: The local language spoken in the health district of Béré.

Nasara: Tchadian Arabic for foreigner, used especially for white foreigners. Not a derogatory term.

N'Djamena: Capital of the Republic of *Tchad,* formerly known as Fort Lamy.

NG tube: Nasogastric tube, a special tube placed through the nose that either carries food and medicine to the stomach or evacuates the contents of the stomach.

Osteomyelitis: infection of the bone, common in developing countries

OR: short for "operating room" where major surgeries are performed in as sterile an environment as possible.

Qahweh: Arabic "coffee", unique for its selection of beans, roasting and addition of other spices like cardamom, cloves, ginger and saffron.

Quincaillerie: Hardware store in French.

Qur'an: the Holy Book of Islam, Arabic "the recitation."

Ramadan: Muslim month-long yearly fast from sunrise to sunset, the end of Ramadan is celebrated with a feast: *Id al-Fitr.* One of the five pillars of Islam.

Salat: Arabic term for the ritual prayer practiced five times daily by devout Muslims. One of the five pillars of Islam.

Shukran: Arabic "thanks" or "thank you."

Symphisiotomy: Obstetrical procedure where the surgeon cuts through the cartilage holding the front of the pelvis together. This effectively widens the pelvic outlet permitting a large baby to be born through a small pelvis.

Tawrat: Arabic "Torah," one of the holy books mentioned by name in the Qur'an. Refers to not only the books of Moses but most of the other books of the Christian Old Testament as well (except the Psalms and other poetry books which are called *az-Zaboor*).

Tchad: One of two recognized English spellings of the sub-Saharan African country bounded by Libya to the north, Sudan to the east, Niger to the West and Nigeria, Central African Republic and Cameroon to the South. The other official and more common spelling is Tchad.

Tchadian Arabic: Second official language of *Tchad*; related to classical Arabic, but a recognized different language. The trade and market language in Tchad.

Vesicle-vaginal fistula: Hole between the vagina and bladder leading to urinary incontinence, usually from a difficult delivery or a complication of a pelvic surgery, often leads to isolation and abandonment in the developing world.

***Xalas!* :** Arabic: "Enough! Okay! All right! At last! Finally! Done!"

Zakat: Arabic for alms for the poor and disadvantaged, an obligation for all Muslims, one of the five pillars of Islam.

ABOUT THE AUTHOR

James Appel, MD graduated from the Loma Linda University School of Medicine in 2000 and then completed a three year residency in Family Practice at the Ventura County Medical Center in California. He spent seven years as the only doctor at the Béré Adventist Hospital directly responsible for the health care of over 150,000 Tchadians. He is the founder of the Moundou Adventist Surgery Center and the Baraka Adventist Hospital Abougoudam. He currently lives in N'Djamena with his wife Sarah and their three children: Miriam, Noah & Isak. When he's not saving lives in Africa he likes to surf, eat Mexican food, run in his five-fingers footwear and talk to Christians positively about Muslims.